ts

Too Big to Be Legal

....

Your Mandated Health Insurance

....

Frank Lobb

Lobb's Analytical Works, LLC
P. O. Box 242
Nottingham, PA 19362

While this book strips our health care system bare to disclose its carefully hidden rationing and illegally inflated bills, it is in no way critical of America's doctors, for they are as much hostages within this fraudulent system as we their patients.

A Word of Appreciation

I would like to thank the following individuals for sharing their insight and knowledge of our health care system. Without their help I could never have connected all the dots. And, while not all of these people were supportive of where I was headed, every one of them contributed to the material in this book.

Joe Pitts	U. S. Congressman & Chair of the House Subcommittee on Health
Dominic Pileggi	Pennsylvania Senator and Leader of the Pennsylvania Legislature
Edwin J. Feulner	President, The Heritage Foundation
Art Hershey	Retired Senior Pennsylvania Representative
Art Caplan	Nationally Acclaimed Bioethicist
Dr. Jane Orient	Executive Director, Association of American Physicians & Surgeons
Linda Peeno	Retired Health Insurance Whistle Blower
David Boaz	Cato Instute
Karl Stark	Philadelphia Inquire
Carl Whitte	Retired Administrator for a large regional hospital
Robert Micheletti	President, Employee Benefit Specialist, Inc
Greg Heller	Attorney; Young, Ricchiuti, Caldwell & Heller
Andrew Schlafly	General Counsel, Association of American Physicians & Surgeons
David Senoff	Attorney; Caroselli, Beachier, McTierman & Conboy
Don McAviney	Fortune 500 Corporate Attorney
Clark Neiley	Constitutional Attorney, Institute for Justice
George Heiney	Attorney; McMichael, Heiney & Sebastian
Joe Roda	Attorney; Roda & Nast
Valerie Gatesman	Attorney, U. S. Department of Labor
Twila Brawley	Citizens Council for Health Freedom
Sue Blevins	Author of Cato Institute's Book, "Medicar's Midlife Crisis
Dr. Fred Himmelstein	Emergency Physician, Jennersville Regional Hospital
Dr. Cecile Pileggi	Physician, Chester County, PA
Ken Woodward	Proofer and Supporter Extraordinaire
Dan Rich	A Touchstone Throughout

Plus a host of other doctors, nurses, health care professionals and interested individuals who shared their time and knowledge. --- **To all of you, a very a sincere <u>Thank You!</u>**

5

Too Big To Be Legal
Your Mandated Health Insurance

ISBN 978-0-615-96299-3

Dedicated in memory of Sandra Lobb and to the support and understanding of Angie Lobb

Contents

__Appendix__

"America's health care system is
neither healthy, caring
nor a system."

Walter Cronkite

Forward

One thing about the U. S. health care system that we should all agree on is that Obamacare (The Affordable Care Act) has made an already all-to complex system an even greater enigma. Constantly attacked from the left and the right with carefully selected talking points, the real issues of health care are lost in the minutia of rancorous partisan talking points. So, let me be clear. This book will not descend into that morass of misdirection, obfuscation, and political-speak where proponents from both sides seek to take us. Fortunately, as with any government program, truth must rest upon well-held points of law for a program to function and survive. Consequently, this book focuses on these points of law — points of law our Washington politicians and the private health care insurance industry are determined to keep hidden — points of law U. S. Congressman Joe Pitts (Chair of the House Subcommittee on Health) was unable to deny, but refuses to disclose — **points of law the U. S. Supreme Court has never been asked to consider** — and, points of law that allow you, an average American, to go around the carefully hidden fraud in Obamacare.

For those of you searching for a way to bring down Obamacare, the book provides a new and unquestionably accurate path to its demise. For those of you simply seeking reasonable health care reform, the book provides a path to responsible negotiations. And, for those of you who simply want to escape the unlawful bills and rationing built into Obamacare, the book provides the path you and your family will need.

While the book leaves the ultimate fix for our broken health care system to others and, unfortunately, our all too cowardly politicians, do not sell this book short. By exposing what can only be deliberate criminal fraud in the unconstitutional marriage of Obamacare with private managed-care health insurance, we create a criminal and civil liability for insurers, employers, and the legal community that cannot be ignored. In essence, rather than being just another book crying over the injustices and excesses in our broken health care system, this book exposes the criminal fraud in the unholy marriage of Obamacare and managed-care health insurance and lays it at the feet of Government, the insurance industry, the legal community and the nation's employers. Furthermore, just like its predecessor, *The Great Health Care Fraud*, the book arms patients with the knowledge they need to access care, coverage and a fair and proper hospital bill regardless of their insurer's efforts to deny these basic rights. And, probably most important, the book describes a new Constitutional challenge to Obamacare that the Government cannot win!

Simply stated, this book takes dead aim at the Government's mandated health insurance with such simplicity, clarity and detail that: 1.) Employers are left no alternative but to disclose the deliberately hidden details of their plans, 2.) Attorneys are made accountable for misrepresenting the details of these plans, 3.) Enrollees are given the knowledge they need to confront the unlawful rationing and fraudulent billing practices inherent in these plans and 4.) Government and the health care insurance industry are left no choice but to seek honest and responsible reform.

Introduction

As a Republican and a strong Conservative when it comes to individual rights under the Constitution, much of the material in this book, as well as my earlier book (*The Great Health Care Fraud*) has been extremely painful to document. Because, rather than support the Constitutional values Conservatives and the Republican Party point to as the bedrock of the party, our leaders have shown themselves more interested in defending the fraud that is inherent in managed-care health insurance. Not to say the Democrats have been any more willing to disclose this travesty. However, the Republican Party is built upon the rights of the individual, and to ignore these rights in pursuit of private market ideology is to surrender our identity, our history and our children's future. Yet that is exactly what the leaders of my party have done. Rather than defend the Constitution, they have turned a blind eye to the clear and deliberate fraud in managed care health insurance.

However, as personal as this issue is for me, the book is not intended to be political in any way. It's simply an analysis of the managed care reality that affects every one of us — Republican and Democrat — Conservative or Liberal. A reality the leaders of both parties have glommed-onto in the hope of reining in the nation's out of control cost of health care.

In this world of ever increasing health care costs, the uncertainty of Obamacare and a never ending call for reform, there is, however, one unarguable truth. The providers of private market health care services (the insurance industry, and our new mega-hospitals) are growing richer by the day at the public's expense. Gone are the family doctors, neighborhood hospitals, local insurance agents, and the systems and bills we could understand. In their place are corporate giants focused on growth and profits rather than service — giants we can't relate to, let alone speak to face to face.

Add to this the fact that while Congress assures us they are working to reduce the cost of health care; they are, in fact, only working to reduce the government's cost of health care. Furthermore, they are doing everything possible to make health care a primary engine of growth for the economy. Whether it's new physical therapy facilities, satellite clinics, regional hospitals or large medical schools; the construction and expansion is explosive and all with the blessing of federal, state, and local governments. Costs you and I will have to shoulder as government and employers shift more and more of the cost of health care onto the individual — an agenda and future that is all too obvious and real. Or, as Steven Brill so aptly wrote in his March 4, 2013 article for Time Magazine, "*a uniquely American gold rush*" is underway in our health care system that will "*put demands on taxpayers to a degree unequalled anywhere else on earth*."

However, for probably the first time in our nation's history, the captains of this gold rush have made a critical mistake. By supporting the marrying of Obamacare with private managed-care health insurance, the insurance industry has put itself within the reach of federal law and the U. S. Constitution. To quote a senior attorney at one of the nation's largest companies, "*They have let the bear into the room*." The bear being the federal courts.

Prior to Obama Care, the regulation of insurance was essentially the sole province of state law. In fact, the courts repeatedly held that all matters involving the regulation of the business of insurance were reserved for the states. However, by mandating that all citizens have health insurance, Obamacare effectively mandates the surrendering of a citizen's right to process and contract in accessing necessary and appropriate health care in that: 1.) Managed care insurance is effectively the only insurance in the market, 2.) All managed-care insurers must include an Enrollee Hold Harmless clause in their provider contracts and 3.) These provider contracts bind essentially every physician, hospital and other provider of health care services in the country. The outcome is inescapable. Obamacare mandates the surrendering of one's doctor-patient relationship and the right to access health care at one's own expense as well as being subjected to a deliberately fraudulent billing system. In short, Obamacare strips individuals of their constitutional right to contract and process as well as opens insurers, hospitals, and employers to a range of federal charges that would appear to be a slam-dunk.

When I wrote the book *The Great Health Care Fraud*, I was obsessed with proving we lose the right to pay for our own health care when we get health insurance from our employer or purchase it directly from a managed-care insurance company. I had spent ten long years pursuing the issue through four courts and was incensed by the lengths the insurance industry and the Commonwealth of Pennsylvania were willing to go to hide the truth — truth I experienced firsthand in the death of my wife, Sandy. As a result, the book became a reflection of my need to set the record straight — to share the proof that had taken me so long to drag out of the insurance industry — to expose what I had come to see as a despicable abuse of power and a complete trashing of the U. S. Constitution.

Unfortunately, the narrow focus of that book left much of the most ingenious fraud of our time untouched — a fact that became increasingly obvious in the countless questions I received since the book was published. This narrow focus has also allowed politicians on both sides of the isle to turn a blind eye to the book and the needs of the American people. As U. S. Congressman Joe Pitts so bluntly put it, *"Why should you care if you can't pay for your own health care."*

Fortunately, the passage of Obamacare changes everything. As my very English wife would say, it gives me a new "whack" at disclosing what is so terribly wrong with our health care system. But, even more important, we all get the opportunity to hold those who are profiting so significantly, from what can only be a deliberate fraud, accountable. Consequently, the goal for this book, and one that I have again promised my wife, Angie, will be my last, is aimed at completely disclosing the fraud in managed care health insurance — to provide a readily available authority for the answers managed-care insurers are determined to keep hidden — and to <u>arm the enrollees in managed-care plans, the medical community, the legal profession, and the advocates for health care reform with the knowledge and</u>

power to hold the insurance industry and their criminal enterprise accountable. In essence, I intend to strip the monster bare and stand it before us without clothes subject to federal law, thanks in large part to Obamacare. However, my number one goal will always be to put the everyday participants in managed-care plans (you, the enrollees, subscribers and beneficiaries in these plans) in a position to obtain their rightful care and coverage regardless of their insurer's decisions on coverage, their employer's fraud, and their politicians' cowardice.

Lastly, let me send a direct challenge to all the politicians, insurance companies, hospitals, large corporate employers, members of the press, and the talking heads of the health care industry that would choose to ignore or dispute the material in this book. You owe the American people a position on this issue. If I am wrong in fact or law, you need only show where and I will celebrate your success in doing what no one has been able to do to date. However, your silence or refusal to engage on this issue can only be the product of blind ideology, greed, or political cowardice. The issue is too important and the proof too overwhelming for there to be any other explanation for silence or obfuscation.

ONE

....

"All health care is personal:"
Dr. Oz

The World of Managed Care

The number of books, reports, papers, and articles dedicated to analyzing the various products and plans in managed-care health insurance is nothing less than mind-blowing — HMO, PPO, POS, MCO, CDH, HDHP, HAS, etc. Yet nowhere in all this mountain of material have I found a single mention of what makes these various acronyms and products one and the same in form and function. In my mind, it's the perfect example of not seeing the forest for the trees.

Yes, HMOs are different from PPOs, and PPOs are different from PSOs, and so on. But each of these products or plans is: 1.) Third-party, 2.) Prepaid, 3.) Operating with provider contracts that have nearly identical terms, conditions, and use of state laws, and 4.) A plan that provides no enrollee ownership. In fact, insurers that offer more than one of these products, which is essentially every major insurer in the country, operate by using a single provider contract that does not differentiate between products.

It's pretty much like attempting to analyze the development of the automobile by sifting through the long history of countless manufacturers, models, colors and accessories while ignoring the basic form and function that characterize all cars — four wheels, a drive train, a transmission, and an engine. In the case of managed-care insurance, these basic elements of form and function are third-party, prepaid care, provider contract, and no enrollee ownership.

An even better example of the point I am making is a contribution I made to drafting the compliance section of the 1992 amendments to the Clean Air Act. The nation was fixated on contentious arguments about the details of exactly what monitoring products should or should not be required by the Act. However, buried in the countless pages of the legislation were just two carefully worded requirements, about six words in total. One was that the monitoring be statistically defensible as continuous, and the other was that it not be presumptively credible under law. That was it. Rather than a contentious process that could only remain lost in a never-ending analysis of product details, we could focus on the two things that defined acceptable monitoring under the Act. In short, industry was free to choose whatever monitoring they preferred as long as it met the two requirements established by Congress. It was a dramatic turnaround for the process and a clear win for form and function over an endless analysis of products and costs.

My point is that once one understands that all the various managed-care products and plans have the same form and function, the world of managed-care health insurance takes on a whole new light. *"The differences between HMO and PPO have blurred,"* and *"a significant majority of consumers do not know which type plan they have,"* and *"comparing competing plans can be difficult even for sophisticated consumers"* because *"important"* information is *"often not available"* (all quotes from The Market Structure of the Health Care Industry, Congressional Research Service Report, April 8, 2010).

Like the vast majority of people in this country, you probably have health insurance and, if so, you most certainly have managed-care health insurance. However, while the name is correct, that's about the only thing you have been led to believe about your insurance that isn't deliberately misleading or false. For instance, it isn't insurance, it is definitely not yours, and it was not created to provide more affordable or higher-quality health care — three indisputable facts. Furthermore, it is not a recent development in the field of health care innovation, and it was certainly not created to rein in the cost of health care. In truth, it's a 1929 product designed by hospitals to serve their needs, not yours or the needs of the nation. Consequently, if we look under the hood, managed-care health insurance has all of the credibility of a 1929 Ford painted to resemble a state-of-the-art 2014 Daytona race car.

The Beginning:

In the early 1900s, people literally either lived or died when they were injured or sick. The health care that was available was only accessible to a privileged few. Furthermore, it was, essentially, limited to avoiding disease, performing only the most basic surgery, extensive nursing care, and a great deal of praying for recovery. However, technology was on the move. Lister had discovered the importance of antiseptics, scientists at Eli Lilly were producing reliable quantities of insulin, and we had a cure for smallpox. We had entered the age of scientific health care. Unfortunately, this new age came with a significant increase in the cost of care. Where hospitalization had cost the average American family 7.6 percent of their total medical expenses in 1918, that figure had risen to thirteen percent by 1929.

Obviously, one cannot mention the year 1929 without addressing the impact of the Great Depression. According to Pulitzer Prize-winning author Paul Starr, "*In just one year after the crash, average hospital receipts per person fell from $236.12 to $59.26.*" This precipitous drop in hospital revenue came on top of the AMA's (American Medical Association) 1927 published concern about "*the inability of people to pay the cost of modern scientific medicine.*" Consequently, the all too real threat of hospital insolvency created by the 1929 crash added to an already growing concern that the rising cost of health care was placing it beyond the reach of the average American family.

It was the perfect storm. The nation's hospitals were facing insolvency, and the AMA had concluded that "*Even among the highest-income group, insufficient care is the rule.*" Furthermore, a story in *The New York Times* declared "*Social Medicine Is Urged in Survey.*" The fallout gave birth to managed care health insurance in the form of what we know today as the Blue Cross Association.

Although there were earlier isolated examples of this new form of health insurance, the perfect storm created by the Great Depression and the ability of what would become the Blue Cross Association to organize hospitals provided the launching pad for today's employer-supplied managed-care health insurance. Hospitals desperately needed a guaranteed source of income, and the American public needed a source of affordable health care. The plans of the future Blue Cross Association fulfilled both needs. Hospitals got the guaranteed payments they needed to remain solvent, and enrollees got a guarantee of all the health care they needed — all for a small monthly or yearly charge or premium.

By charging each participant in a plan (more commonly called an enrollee, subscriber or beneficiary) a small monthly or yearly payment, Blue Cross collected the money they needed to pay the operational costs of the hospitals in their network. And, since Blue Cross collected the money in advance, they paid the hospitals directly. This was exactly the same third-party prepaid health care structure we know today as managed-care health insurance.

We can argue that these plans did not truly prepay for care, because hospitals were paid by a pay-as-you-go system. In other words, hospitals got paid after they delivered care to an enrollee. However, in order to have the money available to pay the hospitals, companies like Blue Cross had to collect their enrollees' payments in advance. Consequently, these companies were, in fact, contract third-party providers of health care services, not insurance companies — a fact Blue Cross originally insisted was the case.

We can also argue that these early plans were not HMOs, PPOs, POSs, MCOs, or any other acronym for a modern-day health care plan. However, such arguments can only serve to obscure the truth. The early plans of Blue Cross had the very same third-party, prepaid, all-necessary-care, no-enrollee-ownership structure of today's managed-care health insurance.

The success of the early Blue Cross plans forced hospitals to organize into networks of hospitals to limit inter-hospital competition. These networks then merged into a single organization known as the American Hospital Association, which adopted the name *Blue Cross Association* in 1939.

Because these early plans were designed by hospitals to benefit hospitals, they covered all hospital expenses right down to the most trivial and inexpensive element of care — all "necessary and appropriate" care. After all, hospitals weren't concerned about controlling the cost of health care; they were focused on getting paid. It's a model for coverage that the market would never allow insurers to change.

By the mid-1930s, the success of prepaid hospital plans, along with the nation's drift toward national health insurance, had physicians worried. They were particularly worried that hospitals would expand their plans into physician services. Physicians reacted by forming their own third-party prepaid plans, which became the Blue Shield Association, which later merged with Blue Cross to form the Blue Cross Blue Shield Association we know today as the Blues.

While we can readily view the history of Blue Cross and Blue Shield as a fight for control of a developing insurance market, it was anything but that. It was simply a fight for control of their respective markets. Because Blue Cross was controlled by hospitals, its focus was on getting their participating hospitals appropriately paid for the services they provided. And because Blue Shield was controlled by doctors, it was focused on getting their doctors appropriately paid.

Others in the private sector were quick to recognize the opportunity being created by the growing market for the Blue Cross Blue Shield plans. However, they were forced to adopt the very same business model. The small monthly payment to a third party for all the health care one might need was simply too popular and well established for anything else to be competitive.

In 1939 just six percent of the U. S. population had any kind of private health insurance for hospitalization. However, by 1941 that number had risen to 12.4 percent of the U. S. population, with fifty-one percent covered by a Blue Cross Blue Shield plan. By 1945 the number had risen to twenty-three percent of the U. S. population, with fifty-nine percent covered by a Blue Cross Blue Shield plan.

Rise of the HMO:

Managed-care plans continued to grow throughout the 1950s and 1960s as individual groups across the country sought to provide affordable health care to their workers or membership. However, the growth lacked the spark needed to make it the national phenomenon we have today. That spark came in 1971 when President Nixon announced a new national health care strategy built on the development of Health Maintenance Organizations or HMOs as they are more commonly known. In truth, this new strategy was simply a new name and acronym for the plans the Blue Cross Blue Shield Association had been supplying since 1929.

Cost containment and coverage for the uninsured had become serious political issues for the Nixon Administration. And, given that Congress had discouraged individuals from purchasing their own health insurance in 1942 by: 1.) making the premiums paid for insurance tax deductible for employers but not for individuals, and 2.) eliminating the private insurance market for those over age 65 by creating Medicare in 1965, the plans offered by the Blue Cross Blue Shield Association offered a readily available private sector solution for the problems the Nixon Administration was facing. Companies had shown themselves willing to supply health insurance as a tax-exempt employee benefit, and Medicare eliminated the cost once an employee retired. Consequently, by making employer-supplied health insurance the focus of the nation's approach to affordable health care, President Nixon sidestepped the growing call for national health insurance and set the nation squarely on a path to a private-sector solution. As a result, President Nixon's new strategy put the full power of the federal government behind the growth of employer-supplied managed care health insurance and assigned

HMOs the primary responsibility for controlling the cost of health care. Nixon's stated goal was to go from thirty HMOs in 1970 to 1,700 by 1976, with forty million enrollees and ninety percent of the population enrolled by 1980. In essence, the race was on.

In 1973 Congress passed the HMO Act, which established Nixon's new strategy as the law of the land. The Act not only provided funding for the development of HMOs, but also required employers with twenty-five or more employees to offer an HMO plan to their employees. Congress gave HMOs an additional boost in 1979 by passing the Employee Retirement Income Security Act (ERISA), which essentially eliminated HMO liability for any denial of coverage or care.

The Role of HMOs in Controlling Costs

By the time Congress passed the HMO Act of 1973, the country had experienced forty years of health insurance that provided all the care a patient needed — forty years of form and function that was devoid of any national effort to curb the cost of health care — forty years of honoring the role of the attending physician in prescribing care — and, forty years of paying for all the "necessary and appropriate" health care enrollees needed and simply adjusting premiums to cover the cost. The passage of the HMO Act in 1973 changed everything.

By passing the HMO Act, Congress not only made HMOs the primary tool for curbing the rising cost of health care, but committed government to supporting the growth of employer-supplied managed-care health insurance. Not coincidentally, insurers immediately began converting to for-profit businesses. Prior to this, the American health care system was comprised largely of nonprofit service organizations. However, the opportunity for growth and profits created by the government's support of HMOs dramatically changed the game. Health care in the United States was forever changed to the profit-driven model that dominates Wall Street and the investment community. As a result, the forty-year model of paying for all the care an enrollee's physician prescribed was placed in direct conflict with the expectations of Congress and the shareholders of the newly created for-profit insurance companies. It was a conflict that would only grow as the nation's nonprofit, service-oriented health care system converted to a market-based, for-profit business model.

Yes, these new for-profit managed-care insurers could pursue profits by negotiating lower rates with their network of doctors and hospitals, but they had been exercising that power for forty years. And, yes they could now negotiate even lower rates because of their greater size and influence. However, there is clearly a law of diminishing returns. Insurers needed something more if they were to deliver the financial performance expected by Congress and demanded by Wall Street. That something could be only the denial of care or, at a minimum, the power to deny the more expensive forms of care and treatment a physician might prescribe. In essence, these new for-profit insurers had to ration care through their own determination of exactly what constitutes "necessary and appropriate" health care. The *"inducement to ration care is the very point of any HMO scheme"* (the U. S. Supreme Court in Pegram et al. v. Herdrich).

It goes without saying that there is no better way for an insurance company, or any company for that matter, to cut costs than to stop paying for things. And that is exactly what HMOs began doing. Doctors were thought to be overprescribing and the determination of "necessary and appropriate" care was subjective, at best. Furthermore, the law requires only that insurers deliver a reasonable average standard of care, not the best or most expensive care available. Therefore, HMOs could continue promoting the forty-year managed-care promise of all "necessary and appropriate" care an enrollee needs, but make their own determination of how to define that term. And that's exactly what they did. They kept the established form and function of managed-care insurance, but made the denial of coverage their primary tool for delivering the financial performance expected by Congress and Wall Street — a practice that grew rapidly *"when big for-profit insurers began to take over,"* as stated in the book *Deadly Spin* by whistleblower Wendell Potter.

Mr. Potter's book provides numerous examples of how far the managed care insurance industry is willing to go in pursuit of peak financial performance. His *firsthand* account of sixteen-year-old Nataline Sarkisyn can bring tears to the eyes of even the strongest of us. Nataline suffered from leukemia, but had essentially beaten the disease. However, the treatments she had received damaged her liver, and without a transplant she would not survive. Doctor after doctor not only prescribed a liver transplant as "necessary and appropriate" care, but pleaded with CIGNA, her insurer, to agree to cover the cost of the operation. CIGNA refused, substituting their own determination of "necessary and appropriate" care for that of the attending physicians. Quoting from Mr. Potter's book, "*The company stood by its decision*" and "*The surgery would not meet CIGNA's definition of medical necessity.*" The end result was that Nataline died while CIGNA worked feverishly to protect its image in the market and steadfastly maintained the transplant was "*outside the scope of CIGNA's coverage*" (again quoted from Wendell Potter's book). Mr. Potter further explains that "*If a critically ill patient dies after an insurance company refuses to pay for a doctor-ordered procedure, which often happens, it can never be proved that the patient would have survived the procedure.*" That is to say, there was no downside for CIGNA in allowing Nataline to die untreated.

Mr. Potter's firsthand account of the internal decision-making of a large insurance company should leave little doubt in anyone's mind that managed-care health insurance in today's world is all about the money. Not coincidentally, the title of Chapter VII in Mr. Potter's book, *Deadly Spin*, is "It's All About the Money."

A Bump in the Road:

While the 1980s and 1990s were a period of unbelievable growth for HMOs and managed-care health insurance, the period also produced a significant bump in the road for the insurance industry as well as for state regulators. Backed by the full weight of the federal government, the growth of HMOs exploded. By 1986, 156 million employees and their dependents were covered by a major medical plan. Unfortunately, explosive growth generally comes with a cost, and it did here as well. By 1989 the overheated insurance market had created a number of unsettling insurer insolvencies, the largest being Maxicare Health Plans. Most troubling was that Maxicare was granted protection under the Federal Bankruptcy Code, which threatened the authority of the states to regulate the health care insurance industry. Equally troubling were the widely reported horror stories of HMOs denying critically needed care which was creating a serious HMO backlash in public opinion. Together, the two issues threatened not only the authority of the states to regulate health insurance but the very structure of the nation's health care system. Surprisingly, however, the states and the insurance industry found themselves on the same page in seeking a solution.

The granting of Chapter 11 protection for Maxicare under the Federal Bankruptcy Code marked a significant departure from what had been the prevailing view of the law because the Federal Bankruptcy Code excludes a "domestic insurance company" from receiving such relief. It's an exception in the law specifically aimed at recognizing the authority of the states to regulate insurance. And, while later court rulings would appear to make the Maxicare decision an exception, the significance of the threat it created for what the states considered their private turf can't be overstated. For, while the Maxicare decision focused on HMOs, it was also applicable to all forms of managed-care health insurance. Furthermore, the reasoning the court used in reaching its decision on Maxicare was inescapable. HMOs and managed-care health plans are not insurance. They are third-party prepaid providers of health care services. This issue has never been fully resolved, which has caused the Norton Institute on Bankruptcy Law to conclude that in the case of HMOs, "*absent an expressed classification under section 109 of the Federal Bankruptcy Code or some federal statute, the classification of an entity should generally follow the law of the state of incorporation, so long as that classification does not frustrate the purpose of the Code.*" This legalese says that managed-care should be ruled insurance if a state says it's insurance. On the other hand, it may *not* be ruled insurance.

While the turmoil that erupted around the Maxicare decision could well be described as a turf war, there was a greater underlying issue. To the states' credit, they and their laws focus on protecting the rights of enrollees rather than the rights of an insurance company or its network of providers. The Federal Bankruptcy Code literally bars any such preferential treatment. In fact, the federal court's ruling in Maxicare described the states' efforts to protect enrollees as *"an anathema to the basic tenant of federal bankruptcy law."* Where state oversight allows a state to quickly shut down an insolvent insurer and transfer the enrollees to another plan, federal bankruptcy bars any such quick resolution of insurer insolvency. Under federal bankruptcy protection, an insolvent insurer is guaranteed the right to largely ignore the needs of its enrollees for months, if not years, while it develops a restructuring plan and submits it to the court for approval.

Fortunately for the states, HMOs only wanted to be viewed as noninsurance businesses in instances of insolvency. That is because there are too many advantages to being an insurance company. For instance, insurance companies are excluded from federal law restricting monopolies — a huge advantage for large insurance companies with regional monopolies.

As for addressing the growing HMO backlash by reining in the power of HMOs to deny coverage and critically needed health care, the states and the insurance industry needed to be on the same page. For, while the public was demanding that the states restrict the power of HMOs to deny coverage, the states couldn't strip HMOs of what Congress viewed as the nation's primary tool for reducing the cost of health care. The logic was inescapable. Congress had created HMOs to negotiate lower costs from providers and <u>eliminate unnecessary and inappropriate care and treatment</u>. Consequently, the only course open to the states and the insurance industry was to find a way to provide the appearance of greater regulation while allowing HMOs to continue denying coverage outside the view of the public.

A Model Set in Concrete:

The solution that both the states and the insurance industry needed came in the form of an HMO Model Act drafted by the National Association of Insurance Commissioners' (NAIC) in the early 1990s. This model piece of legislation was adopted state by state across the entire country to provide a unified approach to the problems HMOs were creating. NAIC is the U. S. standard-setting and regulatory support organization governed by the insurance commissioners from the fifty states, the District of Columbia, and the five U. S. territories. Its published mission is to: 1.) Protect the public interest; 2.) Promote competitive markets; 3.) Facilitate fair and equitable treatment of insurance customers; 4.) Promote the reliability, solvency, and financial solidity of insurance institutions; and 5.) Support and improve state regulation of insurance. Simply stated, NAIC is the national organization for state-based insurance regulation.

While the form and function of managed-care health insurance hadn't changed appreciably since its inception in 1929, the changes in state law brought on by Maxicare and NAIC's HMO Model Act set this form and function in concrete as well as made it sustainable. After all, the backlash of the 1990s had clearly proven that it's one thing for insurers to have the power to ration health care and quite another to exercise that power under the critical eye of the public.

Simply put, the states' adoption of NAIC's HMO Model Act gave insurers the power to continue rationing care, but under a fog of misleading definitions, appeal procedures, and state laws and regulations. Heralded as a way to protect enrollees from insurer insolvency and the denial of "necessary and appropriate" health care, the provisions actually reinforce the states' authority to regulate insurance while guaranteeing HMOs the authority to continue rationing care by denying doctors, hospitals, and other providers of health care services any compensation whatsoever unless they accept the insurer's decision on "necessary and appropriate" health care. In other words, by creating a host of new requirements for

HMOs the states conveyed the impression they were protecting enrollees. However, outside the view of the public they guaranteed these insurance companies the right to continue denying care and treatment through secret provider contracts with essentially every doctor, hospital and provider of health care services in the country. In essence, they set the form and function of managed-care and the industry's ability to ration health care in concrete. Consequently, the only way your doctor or hospital can provide the "necessary and appropriate" care your insurer refuses to approve is to provide it free of charge, <u>even if you are ready, willing, and able to write a check to cover the cost</u>. This is the law in every state in the country.

Best known as the Enrollee Hold Harmless clause, it's a mandated provision in the provider contract that insurers are required to have with every in-network doctor, hospital, and other providers of health care services (essentially every provider of health care services in the country). Independence Blue Cross of southeastern Pennsylvania, alone, advertises over fifty-five thousand such in-network doctors under contract.

Furthermore, while the letter of these state laws would appear to cover only HMOs, the enforcement of these laws allows for no differentiation between HMOs, PPOs, PSOs, or any other form of managed-care health insurance. The *"Differences between plans have blurred over the last two decades"* and *"HMO and PPO plans no longer occupy distinct market segments"* (*The Market Structure of the Health Insurance Industry, Congressional Research Service*, 2010). Insurers are completely free to gather all their various acronyms and managed-care health insurance plans under a single provider contract. And they do exactly that to create a universal business model beyond the view of the public and the enrollees in their plans. It's a model specifically designed to strip enrollees of their right to due process and contract in their relationship with their in-network doctors, hospitals, and the other providers of health care services. And, it's a model that cannot be recast or reformed without completely rewriting the health care laws of every state and the millions of secret provider contracts between insurers and their in-network doctors, hospitals, and other providers of health care services.

The fact that so little is known about the NAIC HMO Model Act and its Enrollee Hold Harmless clause should come as no surprise. For, while the Act and the Enrollee Hold Harmless clause form the most important element in the design of the managed-care business model, it's one that can't survive the light of day.

By requiring doctors, hospitals, and all the other in-network providers of health care services to contractually accept nonpayment for any "necessary and appropriate" care that an insurer refuses to approve, insurers can deny providers any payment whatsoever unless they accept the insurer's decision on what <u>a patient should or should not receive</u>. This is the core of what we know today as managed-care health insurance and <u>the only game in town</u>.

> <u>Note</u>: While I have chosen to use *necessary and appropriate* care for this book, *medical necessity*, *necessary and appropriate*, and *reasonable and necessary* are all terms used by the insurance industry for determining coverage. I've chosen to use *necessary and appropriate* for the book simply to standardize on a term and because it's the version I most often encountered throughout my research and years of litigation. Furthermore, the courts have viewed these various determinations of coverage as one and the same.

Two

....

*"Whenever a doctor cannot
do good, he must be kept
from doing harm."*
Hippocrates

My Introduction to Managed Care

My introduction to the hidden world of managed-care health insurance came with a heavy price — the death of my first wife, Sandra Sargisson Lobb, or simply Sandy, as so many of us called her. I told this story in my first book, so I won't repeat it here. What I will do is to stress that we were a family like the vast majority in this country that simply assumed that the health insurance we get from our employer will be there when we need it. We also assumed that we could purchase any care our insurance failed to provide from our family doctor or the hospitals in our area. And of course we never doubted the trust and confidence we placed in our family doctor.

All this changed when our insurance company denied Sandy the hospital care her doctor insisted she needed. But that was only the beginning of my education. The real zinger came when the hospital told me that the contract they had with our insurer prevented them from allowing me to pay for Sandy's care. In other words, the insurer not only refused to pay for the care Sandy needed, but their provider contract barred the hospital from allowing me to pay for it. The bottom line is that Sandy died while I sputtered and fumed over how an insurance company could prevent me from paying for Sandy's care, not only at our local hospital but at all the hospitals I contacted. What made the situation even worse was that everyone I spoke to in the health care industry and government lied about what was happening. I was clearly being denied the right to pay for Sandy's care, and I had pushed the issue to the point where there was no mistaking what they had told me. At the same time, everyone I went to for help outside the hospitals insisted that no such refusal was possible — that there was nothing that could possibly prevent me from paying for Sandy's care.

At the time, the only rational explanation I could think of was that Sandy's insurance company had created a practice that was outside the law and was enforcing it through secrecy and pure economic power. After all, Sandy's insurer was reported to control over seventy percent of the revenue that hospitals received in our area of Pennsylvania. They literally owned the health insurance market. I couldn't conceive of such an abuse of power extending beyond Sandy's insurer.

This marked the beginning of what would become my long pursuit of the truth behind what had cost Sandy her life and what I argue is the greatest fraud in my lifetime and quite possibly our nation's history. Furthermore, it's a fraud that no one of consequence wants disclosed — my conclusion after an educational process that at times took my breath away.

The insurance companies don't want it disclosed because it is the core of their power to ration health care, something that has the potential to unleash a rash of class-action lawsuits the industry cannot survive without significant reform. The states don't want it disclosed because they created the system in order to retain the authority to regulate insurance. The federal government doesn't want it disclosed because it could disrupt the nation's entire health care system. The hospitals don't want it disclosed because it would expose them to all kinds of liability. The doctors can't disclose it without exposing themselves to retribution that could destroy their ability to practice. The Republican leadership, and certainly leading conservatives, can't disclose it because private managed-care health insurance is their creation and their alternative to the left's single-payer system. The leadership of the Democratic Party can't disclose it because it would threaten the survival of employer-supplied health insurance. And, most surprising of all, the long list of people and organizations that advocate for consumer protection, health care reform, and so many other righteous causes won't disclose it because it would damage their business, i.e., the very profitable business of advocating for people willing to contribute to health care reform. It's a reality that took me more than ten long, hard years to get through my thick skull — a reality that dawned on me only when all my many expressions of outrage over what had happened to Sandy were swept aside by these folks like puffs of smoke on a windy day.

Organizations and individuals like Consumer Watchdog, U. S. Senator John McCain, the American Medical Association, Cato Institute, The Heritage Foundation, Americans for Democratic Action, U. S. Representative Joe Pitts, Chair of the House Subcommittee on Health, U. S. Senator Robert Casey, AARP, The Institute for Justice, and the ACLU all listened and then simply went away. Yet not one of these organizations or people offered a single point of disagreement on a fact or point of law that I describe in my book *The Great Health Care Fraud*. To quote the constitutional attorney for one of these groups, "*You are not hearing me. I'm not saying I disagree with you. I'm saying we just don't want to deal with it*."

Unfortunately, I was taught by my grandfather that "*If there is a will, there is a way*." Furthermore, I honestly believed that no one could deny that we had been prevented from paying for the care Sandy needed. After all, I had dealt with so many people and the refusals had been so direct and clearly stated. And, who could ever claim that refusing to allow me to pay for Sandy's care was an acceptable practice for an insurance company? It all seemed so simple — simple enough to launch me down a road of ten years of litigation through four separate courts in pursuit of just one thing: the truth behind the façade of all the "necessary and appropriate" care

<u>you will ever need</u> and the power of an insurance company to deny access to health care even when we are willing to pay for it with our own money. *"You are to be congratulated for your perseverance on this issue as well as for the publication of your book,"* Edwin J. Feulner, president of The Heritage Foundation, stated to me in a personal letter dated May 31, 2012. See Appendix 4.

I won't bore you with the rest of my story because it would contribute little to the focus of this book. Or stated more directly, why and how I got the material and understanding for the book is of little importance. In fact, if I were to retell the story of Sandy and our family's ten years of frustrating litigation, I could rightly be said to be obsessing over things that happened years in the past rather than what this book is about. So please, let my bullheaded pursuit of the truth about managed-care health insurance and what has been so carefully and deliberately hidden from the American people define me and this book. For while what happened to Sandy is a tragedy, her death needs to be seen as merely a catalyst for exposing a far greater wrong that extends to millions of unsuspecting Americans. We need to focus on the carefully constructed fraud that is managed-care health insurance and robs every one of us of this country's promise of individual liberty and freedom. For nothing can be more American than our right to freely access and contract for the health care we need for ourselves and the families we love.

I will add only that over my long years of frustrating litigation and the constant stream of motions and replies, the attorneys for the two insurance companies and the Commonwealth of Pennsylvania proved they were far better litigators than yours truly. In fact, I am one hundred percent sure they will tell you they won every hearing and successfully defended every charge. However, during those many proceedings, these same attorneys were forced to reveal, bit by bit, the details of their system — details that I can assure you they did not want disclosed, details that I can now share with you and the public. So unless I am missing something, this naïve and untrained litigator obtained what he and the Lobb family sought from the very beginning.

While the court records will never show us winning a single

motion or hearing, this book provides all the proof I and my family will ever need for determining who won those cases. It discloses the details of a system that even the insurance industry cites as a violation of federal law — details that can ensure you never face the denial of critical health care as we did with Sandy — details that can guarantee you get the care, coverage, and uninflated billing you and your family deserve.

In summary, I admit that I couldn't have been more naïve in my pursuit of justice. I filed against the wrong party, made the wrong charges, expected support where there was none, and failed to recognize the importance of the issue to both the insurance industry and government as a whole. I simply couldn't have been more wrong. Nevertheless, as Philadelphia hockey fans know only too well, *"The game is never over until the fat lady sings."* And it's my firm belief that the facts in this book will prove that power and money can't drive truth off the ice to end the game.

THREE

*"Many a small thing has
been made large by the right
kind of advertising:"*
                                        Mark Twain

The Plan They Promote

We can't go anywhere today without being exposed to an advertisement for health insurance in magazines, on TV, on our car radio, and on the well-placed billboards we pass every day on the way to work. All are dedicated to showing us the miracles of modern-day health care that are readily available from an insurer's health plan. Enhanced by the finest of today's computer graphics, text, and sound, these advertisements constantly assure us of plans that are carefully designed to meet our every need. And, I defy you or anyone to show me an insurer that doesn't claim to provide the most affordable, informative, reliable, and highest-quality health care that modern technology can provide. You *"can make better health care decisions with our guidance"* (Cigna Health Group); We are *"always here when you need us"* (Kaiser Permanente); *"Humana helps you put your needs first"* (Humana Health Insurance); *"The most admired health insurance"* (Aetna); *"The best combination of health care and value"* (Wellpoint Inc.); *"Live fearlessly"* (Independence Blue Cross); and on and on.

While these promotions are obviously aimed at you and the

rest of the general public, they are, in truth, little more than window dressing for a product that is primarily sold to employers in closed-door meetings focused on cost and efficiency. Quoting the report from the 2006 National Conference on Efficiency in Health Care, the "*skyrocketing cost of health care is not sustainable if employers are to continue insuring employees*" and "*there is a perception that the lack of efficiency is driving unnecessary costs in health care*" and "*There is increasing pressure for employers to measure efficiency.*"

The simple truth is that insurers have to sell their plans to two very different groups. The first and foremost group is comprised of the nation's employers, who purchase the overwhelming majority of health insurance in the country. The second audience is comprised of the employees who receive this insurance but have a very different perspective on quality, cost, and efficiency (once again a conclusion of the 2006 National Conference on Efficiency in Health Care). As a result, insurers aggressively promote a vision of "your" plan, "your" doctor, and "guaranteed access" to the finest health care to enrollees while they simultaneously promise employers in closed-door meetings the lowest possible cost by limiting access to only the most cost-effective care.

Two audiences, two very different messages — "All the very highest quality care an enrollee will ever need" to the folks who will have to depend on the insurance for, literally, life itself and "Only the most cost-efficient care" to the employers who purchase the plans. It's an example of the old bait-and-switch ploy at its finest.

The bottom line is that insurers go to great lengths to describe their plans as providing: 1.) our very own health plan, 2.) our doctor, 3.) the highest possible quality, 4.) full transparency, and 5.) an insurance product designed to meet our every health care need. In short, what more could we want?

FOUR

....

*"Fraud and falsehood only
dread examination.
Truth invites it:"*
Samuel Johnson

The Plan They Don't Want Us to See

The easiest way to explain why managed-care insurers refuse to disclose key provisions in their plans is to compare managed-care health insurance with automobile insurance. At first glance one could reasonably assume that both forms of insurance serve the same purpose, i.e., to protect individuals from unexpected but necessary costs. In the case of health insurance, the unexpected but necessary costs are for the care and treatment needed to return an enrollee to full health. In the case of automobile insurance, the unexpected but necessary costs are for the care and treatment needed to return an automobile to its undamaged condition. Therefore, both forms of insurance have the same need to limit coverage to "necessary and appropriate" services and costs. However, this is where life gets far more difficult for a health-care insurance company.

While both forms of insurance have to limit coverage to "necessary and appropriate" services and costs, only the automobile insurer is free to determine what those services and costs are for a particular claim. The automobile insurer simply sends its adjuster into a body shop to inspect the damaged vehicle and decide exactly what will and will not be done to repair the damage. By contrast, the health care insurer has no such freedom. The laws of every state reserve the determination of "necessary and appropriate" health care to a properly licensed attending physician (typically your doctor). A physician who cannot be a direct employee of a health-care insurance company. Furthermore, the automobile insurer is only required to return a damaged vehicle to its pre-accident condition, and the cost cannot exceed the fair market value of a similar undamaged vehicle.

Health care insurance companies face a far more challenging reality. Here the goal must always be to return a patient to "full" health, regardless of the age or condition of the patient, and only the attending physician can decide what is needed. Furthermore, under the laws of every state, once treatment is begun, it must be continued until it's either complete or no longer of value. However, the most important difference between these two forms of insurance is the health care insurer's inability to establish what needs to be done to treat a particular patient. That's because "necessary and appropriate" health care has proven to be *notoriously difficult, if not impossible, to define*" (*The Futility of Medical Necessity*, E. Haavi Morreim, University of Tennessee, 2001) and "*when it comes to selecting the appropriate level of care, medical necessity trumps everything else*" (*A Refresher on Medical Necessity*, Peter R. Jensen, MD, CPC, 2006). Consequently, the laws of every state assign the authority for determining "necessary and appropriate" health care to the attending physician, not a health care insurance company. In other words, while an automobile insurer is free to make an absolute determination of what is needed to repair a damaged vehicle, the health care laws of every state assign that absolute authority to an outside and traditionally independent attending physician (your doctor).

Unfortunately, while the law may be on the side of an enrollee and his or her doctor for determining "necessary and appropriate" health care, we have all heard far too many reports of enrollees' being denied coverage for care that has been prescribed by their doctor — far too many reports of insurer's simply overruling a doctor to limit coverage — far too many stories of insurers' denying coverage in order to reduce the cost of care. And, may I say it? Far too many stories of insurers rationing lifesaving care over the strenuous objections of an enrollee's doctor.

So, how can managed-care insurers circumvent the law? How can they substitute their business judgment on "necessary and appropriate" health care for the medical judgment of an attending physician, your doctor? How can they ignore an enrollee's right to receive the care prescribed by his or her doctor and approve only a less expensive standard of care? The answer is that they simply don't allow the public, particularly enrollees, to see the details of their health plans. *"My gut tells me that the PR nightmare wouldn't be worth the problems an explicit cost-effectiveness criterion might entail"* for limiting coverage (Judy Wagner of the Congressional Office of Technology Assessment, National Symposium On Medical Necessity, Apr. 1995). Or, to say it more simply, they deliberately hide the details of their plans.

"Do not be fooled when the health insurance industry claims that it has abandoned its old practices" of denying care and *"private health insurance is a labyrinth of misleading terms of art designed to help companies minimize coverage and maximize profits"* (Congressional testimony of whistleblowers Dr. Linda Peeno and Wendell Potter, respectively, September 16, 2009). Both of these people are accomplished professionals who served at the highest level within the insurance industry. They have seen firsthand the practices and policies the managed-care insurance industry deliberately hide.

(A) It's Not Your Plan:
"Individuals with health insurance do not own or control those policies in the same way that they own and control auto insurance, homeowners' or life insurance. For most Americans their employers own the policy" (Edwin J. Feulner, President of The

Heritage Foundation, May 31, 2012). *"Until you pointed it out, I would have thought I owned my plan"* (retired judge Harry J. Farmer, Oct. 2013).

To own something, one needs to have a bill of sale, a contract, policy, or some form of signed document demonstrating ownership. Enrollees in managed-care health plans have none of these because they do not own what they have been led to view as "their" very own plan and insurance. Where automobile insurance, homeowners' insurance, and life insurance companies provide an insured individual with a detailed and enforceable contract or policy, managed-care health insurance provides enrollees with no such enforceable rights or contract. In the vast majority of cases, employers simply allow their qualified employees to access the employer's health plan as part of an employee benefit package. And where an enrollee purchases a plan directly, the insurer simply allows the enrollee to access the benefits contained in the insurer's plan.

To illustrate just how far insurers are willing to go to encourage enrollees to view managed-care plans as their own personal insurance, consider the following. Since enrollees have no ownership in their employer's health plan, they lack the right to sue an insurer for breach of contract. After all, if there is no contract, there can be no breach of contract and no duty owed to an enrollee. Consequently, the only party that can owe a duty to an enrollee who gets his or her health insurance form an employer is the employer. Even so, insurers have shown themselves surprisingly willing to be the defendant in breach of contract suits rather than simply pursue summary judgment based on the lack of enrollee ownership in the plan. In my case, this willingness to accept the role of defendant lasted the better part of ten years. So while I can only guess at why Sandy's insurer was so willing to subject itself to years of costly litigation, I have to believe it was for two reasons: 1.) Insurers want enrollees to view these plans as their very own so they don't sue employers that are the highly valued customer of an insurer and 2.) Insurers do not want to redirect these suits to employers that lack both the knowledge and willingness to defend the insurer's policies, actions and <u>masterful fraud</u>.

For absolute proof of just who owns these health plans we need only look at the law. In order to protect the rights of employees, Congress passed the Retiree Employment Income Security Act (ERISA) in 1979. The Act not only makes employers directly responsible for their health plans, but makes their management of these plans a fiduciary duty owed to the employees who are enrolled in these plans.

The bottom line is that you do not own your managed-care health insurance or plan. The insurance industry and your employer just want you to believe you do because it greatly simplifies their world.

(B) It's Not Even Insurance:

As shown earlier in the book, managed-care health plans are not an insurance product but a third-party pre-purchase of the future health care needs of its enrollees. That's why managed-care health insurance is insurance in name only. So whenever an enrollee's doctor prescribes what he or she believes is "necessary and appropriate" care, the care has actually been paid for in advance. However, managed-care insurers cannot afford to have enrollees see it that way as it would create far too many problems. Instead, enrollees are led to believe that their plan is an insurance product where coverage is guaranteed by the terms and conditions of their policy, i.e., their plan. But enrollees have no policy, contract or any enforceable rights to terms and conditions that define coverage. Enrollees are simply left to trust that the care they will receive will be the same best-available "necessary and appropriate" health care that the insurer promotes rather than the rationed product they choose to deliver and hide.

(C) Not Your Doctor:

If you sued your health-care insurance company for breach

of contract and then discovered that your attorney had a secret contract with the insurer, it would be a very big deal. You would have every right to demand a mistrial, sue the attorney for malpractice, and insist that the bar association strip the attorney of his or her license to practice law. It's a conflict of interest in the attorney-client relationship that the judicial system will not tolerate. Unfortunately, the enrollees in managed-care health plans face this same conflict of interest when they consult with what they are led to believe is "their" doctor and "their" doctor-patient relationship — a relationship that is well held to embody the same reliance, faith, confidence, and fiduciary duty that exists in the attorney-client relationship.

For those who question my use of the word *secret* when referring to the contracts that all in-network physicians have with managed-care insurers, you only need ask your doctor, insurer, or state department of insurance for a copy of your doctor's provider contract and then stand back and watch the dance. Furthermore, there is a test the IRS uses to establish the actual employer in complex contractual relationships that sheds light on whether an insurer can rightfully claim that their in-network doctor is "your" doctor. It's called the "Same Desk Principle." In essence, the test looks for where an individual gets direction and management and who controls the actual work product as opposed to who actually writes the check to compensate the individual. I submit that any reasonable interpretation of an in-network physician's secret provider contract, using the IRS's Same Desk Principle, verifies that in-network physicians are the insurer's doctors and not an enrollee's or yours. After all, the only way what is supposedly "your" doctor can get paid is to provide the care that the insurer decides is appropriate.

(D) Different Covered Services:

As much as the insurance industry would like us believe that Covered Services in a managed-care health plan are the services an insurer approves and pays for, *they are not*. In fact, Covered Services, by law, precedent, and contract, are the services *available* in a managed-care plan, regardless of whether or not an insurer agrees to approve and pay for them in a particular instance. While this might seem a trivial point, I assure you it is not. It is a widely held misunderstanding that robs enrollees of their rights and distorts the entire process of accessing "necessary and appropriate" health care. Even worse, it's a misunderstanding that is actively encouraged by the insurance industry as a way to circumvent the law, overrule the decisions of an attending physician, and hide the meaning of a state-mandated Enrollee Hold Harmless clause that must be included in every contract that insurers are required to have with their in-network doctors, hospitals, and other providers of health care services.

Let's take a closer look at the term, Covered Services. Let's look at why the insurance industry, along with the state insurance agencies, are so anxious to have litigants mistakenly pursue issues of coverage rather than an insurer's refusal to provide the care that has been promised, properly prescribed, and paid for in advance. Let's examine why a term that is so well understood within the insurance industry and state governments can be so misunderstood by enrollees and the public.

Because managed-care was originally created to provide guaranteed payments to doctors and hospitals, it wasn't until Congress passed the 1973 HMO Act that managed-care insurers felt the need to limit the overall cost of health care. While the early managed-care plans received discounted rates from doctors and hospitals, their focus was on ensuring that their network of doctors and hospitals got appropriately paid for everything they did. After all, these early managed-care insurers were run by doctors and hospitals for the benefit of doctors and hospitals. Furthermore, the predominant form of employer-supplied health insurance in 1973 was indemnity insurance that also covered essentially everything an attending physician prescribed. Consequently, President Nixon's new name for managed-care health insurance (HMOs) faced a real quandary. HMOs were being asked to win over the majority of the nation's workers and providers while curtailing what both could receive from this new form of employer-supplied health insurance. In addition, the country was entering a period where the expansion of employee benefits was an economic reality. Employees were both expecting and getting more, not less. In essence, HMOs were being asked to become the dominant form of health insurance in the country while reversing themselves on the very thing that had made managed-care plans so successful, i.e., paying for all the care a doctor prescribed.

So how does one market a product that delivers less than what consumers are used to receiving and less than what they want? How does one successfully market a product that delivers less than the competition? Normally, one simply offers the product at a lower price and claims a higher value for the money spent. But the consumers in this case were not the ones actually paying for the insurance. The nation's employers were.

The obvious answer is one all Americans know only too well. It's called bait-and-switch. The seller simply promises what the consumer wants to hear, but uses the fine print in the deal to deliver a less costly product. And that is exactly what HMOs did. By introducing the term *medical necessity* in the fine print of their obligation to pay for Covered Services, HMOs gave everyone the impression they were still promising all the care an attending physician prescribed. However, in closed-door meetings with employers and government, they were free to promise an unrelenting assault on the cost of care through the elimination of what insurers viewed as unnecessary costs and services — an assault that would lead to the HMO backlash of the 1990s.

In truth, the insurers' strategy was actually quite ingenious. By introducing the concept of "medical necessity" in the definition of Covered Services, insurers were able to assure enrollees and their doctors that nothing was changing. After all, the laws of every state mandated that this determination could only be made by a properly licensed *attending* physician. A physician's review of a patient's medical records "*does not meet the requirement of a physical examination or establish a legitimate practitioner-patient relationship*" (New York State Board for Professional Medical Conduct, 2007). Furthermore, the definition of *medical necessity* is so

46

vague that no one could be expected to discern a meaningful change in coverage. Medical necessity *"invites enrollees to entertain high and uniform expectations"* ("The Futility of Medical Necessity," *Health & Medicine*, 2001). And, *"It is practically impossible to write contractual terms that precisely define a patient's entitlement to care"* ("Consumers Versus Managed Care," Clark C. Havighurst, July 2001).

In my mind, there really can't be a better example of bait-and-switch. Enrollees had no ability to understand the significance of the introduction of *medical necessity* into the definition of Covered Services. In fact, that is exactly why enrollees, and generations before them, looked to *their* doctor for skill and counseling. Similarly, why would doctors understand the significance of this new term when the laws of every state assigned this very determination to them and only them?

It is this stark difference between the perceived promise of Covered Services and the Covered Services an insurer intends to honor that has doctors sitting squarely in the center of our broken health care system and <u>makes the managed-care business model legally indefensible</u>. On one hand, managed care actively promotes the breadth of their Covered Services and access to the highest standard of care science can provide. However, when they deny coverage or insist on a less expensive course of treatment, they claim it's an appropriate contractual determination of Covered Services under the terms and conditions of the enrollee's plan. They insist it is not the medical determination that it most certainly is and they cannot make under the laws of every state in the country. In short, their definition of Covered Services is deliberately different from what they would have enrollees and the nation believe.

For those needing additional proof of this deliberate misrepresentation, please refer to my earlier book, *The Great Health Care Fraud*. In it I go to great lengths to document what can be viewed only as deliberate misrepresentation and fraud by both the insurance industry and the state departments of health and insurance.

The bottom line is that the managed-care insurance industry

uses two very different definitions for the term Covered Services. When insurers promote their plans, they actively encourage a belief that Covered Services constitutes ALL the "necessary and appropriate" care your doctor prescribes. However, when they deny coverage or insist on a less expensive course of treatment, insurers claim they have the contractual right to overrule your doctor and apply their own determination of "necessary and appropriate care." All the "necessary and appropriate" care your doctor, by law, determines in order to sell their plan. Only the "necessary and appropriate" care the insurer determines when providing actual coverage.

Later sections in the book will have a great deal more to say about the deliberate use of these two very different definitions of Covered Services.

(E) Hidden Restrictions on Emergency Care:

Several years ago I awoke from a deep sleep to find my wife laboring for breath and in serious trouble. Because it was the middle of the night, I rushed her to the emergency room at the nearest hospital, only to be once again confronted by the plan that insurers refuse to disclose.

Since we had three separate and overlapping health plans, I wasn't the least bit concerned about the cost of her care. I simply assumed that the emergency care promised by our plans and the duty a doctor owes to a patient had us all on the same page. Unfortunately, I could not have been more mistaken. Contrary to what managed-care plans promote, the reality of available emergency services is quite different.

What we are not told is that when an enrollee is admitted to a hospital for emergency care, the hospital is required to assign a single code that defines the emergency — a code that determines exactly how much the hospital will be paid regardless of whether it takes one day or one hundred days to treat the patient. That's right, one price regardless of how long it takes to "successfully" treat an enrollee. One price that is specifically designed to limit the care that is provided as well as encourage a quick discharge back to the street.

The result is that hospitals and their emergency room doctors have become experts at classifying an emergency as one they can quickly remedy (better stated as "stabilize") and allow for a quick discharge. For example, say an enrollee is admitted to a hospital emergency room for severe stomach cancer. One would reasonably expect that the code assigned to the emergency would be for stomach cancer. At this point, I hope you are not going to be surprised to learn that this is absolutely _not_ true. Instead, the enrollee will almost certainly be admitted for gastrointestinal discomfort, stabilized to reduce pain, and then quickly discharged back to the street.

In the case of my wife, I realized something was wrong and demanded her emergency be defined as a life-threatening heart condition which required that she be formally admitted to the hospital. Once admitted, she received the care and in-hospital time she needed. However, I have no doubt what-so-ever that had I not insisted on the emergency being properly defined, she would have been quickly discharged with a mere assurance that her discomfort had been addressed and told to see a doctor as soon as possible.

Should you find yourself or a loved one in an emergency room, ask to see the results of their diagnosis and whether a doctor has signed it. Insist that a physician sign an order for discharge. And, watch the consternation that this will create as it never happens. Consequently, insurers get to limit the cost of the emergency care while ensuring a quick discharge back to the street. And, the hospital gets to escape responsibility for failing to properly treat the patient.

(F) Rationing for Lower Costs and Higher Profits:

No one can reasonably dispute the fact that managed-care

insurers ration health care in pursuit of lower costs and higher profits. The *"inducement to ration care is the very point of any H.M.O. scheme"* and *"No H.M.O. organization could survive without some incentive connecting physician reward with treatment rationing"* and *"the profit incentive to ration care"* goes *"to the very point of any H.M.O. scheme"* (all quotes from Justice David H. Souter, U. S. Supreme Court decision in Pegram et al. v. Herdrich, 2000). However, it is equally true that managed-care insurers view the term *rationing* as one that must be avoided at all costs. *"H.M.O.'s make decisions weighing costs against benefits. Justice Souter called that rationing, but there are other ways to talk about* it" (Karen M. Ignagni, president of the American Association of Health Plans, *The New York Times*, June 18, 2000). Justice Souter *"did not understand the use of the word ration. It's an unfortunate word, which implies that needed care is being cut back. I'd call it changing the incentives, or changing the site of care, as medically appropriate"* (Alan D. Bloom, senior vice president and general counsel of Maxicare Health Plans, www.consumerwatchdog.org). *"Among H.M.O.'s the very word rationing is radioactive because it suggests that some patients are denied treatments they need"* — ("Wake up, America" (M. Gregg Bloche, Georgetown University Law Center, *The New York Times*, June 18, 2000). And, we need to be more *"up front in talking to patients about rationing"* (Dr. Steven D. Pearson, director of The Center for Ethics in Managed Care, Harvard Medical School).

All this is a bit like the subject of premarital sex when I was growing up. So long as it wasn't discussed, we could all pretend it wasn't happening. However, premarital sex didn't have a three trillion-dollar industry committed to keeping the subject hidden nor was it something we all depend on for literally our right to life itself.

The unfortunate truth is that rationing is a fundamental part of every form of managed-care health insurance (HMO, PPO, POS, etc.). It's an indisputable fact. It's also an indisputable fact that the managed-care insurance industry desperately wants to avoid acknowledging it. But the real travesty is the industry's refusal to disclose how it applies and enforces rationing in plans that we have to accept on blind faith.

(G) Secret Provider Contracts:

As committed as the managed-care industry is to avoiding any mention of rationing, it has been loud and consistent in warning us of the rationing that will occur from any additional involvement by the federal government in our health care system. The industry's clear but unstated message is that private plans _do not ration health care_. However we know that they do. So how can the insurance industry live in these two very opposite worlds? How can we have the Supreme Court ruling that rationing is _"very point of any HMO scheme"_ on one hand and the public largely believing that rationing is something we only need fear from further government involvement in our health care? How can insurers make rationing _"the very point"_ of a managed- care plan, but do so outside the view of the public and the press? Even more to the point, how can insurers enforce their rationing when common sense and the law tell us that only our doctor can determine the care that we need and have been promised by our health plan?

They do it by establishing secret contracts with every doctor, hospital, and other provider of health care services in their network of approved providers — contracts that define every element of the provider's relationship with the insurer — contracts that contain terms and conditions that limit an enrollee's right to coverage — contracts that place strict and enforceable limits on the ability of an attending physician (your doctor) to determine the "necessary and appropriate" health care you or any other enrollee can receive — contracts with limits that cannot be found in any information that is available to an enrollee. Most importantly, these are contracts that clearly and irrevocably sever what you, or any reasonable person, would assume is his or her personal, private and legally protected doctor-patient relationship. And, they are contracts that are state-reviewed, state-approved, and held as public documents. However, they are locked away from the public and never explained or even acknowledged.

For those who doubt the degree of secrecy attached to these contracts, please consider the following references.

Congressional Research Service, 1997

The Congressional Research Service's report for Congress entitled "Managed Health Care: Federal and State Regulation," issued in 1997, is more than thirty pages long. Yet it states only that the *"contracts between an HMO and a participating provider be in writing"* and that *"The HMO must ensure that in the event that it fails to pay for services, the subscriber or enrollee is not liable to the provider for any amounts owed by the HMO."* The report provides no further explanation of a provision in state-mandated contracts that any first-year law student would recognize raises all kinds of questions. It's an omission that can only be intentional.

Congressional Research Service, 2010

A second Congressional Research Service report in 2010 entitled A second Congressional Research Service report in 2010 entitled "The Market Structure of the Health Insurance Industry" is more than sixty pages long. Yet it makes absolutely *no* mention of how these state-mandated provider contracts are used to ration health care by requiring providers to supply only the care that an insurer has decided is medically "necessary and appropriate." Furthermore, the report fails to even mention the issues that this universal contract language has to create.

NAIC HMO Model Act, revised July 2005

The Act says that managed care's provider contracts shall be treated as *"trade secrets or privileged or confidential"* commercial information.

The American Medical Association, 2005

The AMA's "Model Managed Care Contract," published in 2005, is sixty-seven pages long and is intended to both explain and recommend every element that a doctor must consider before signing one of these state-mandated provider contracts. However, section 3.11 of this "Model Contract," a section entitled "Sole

Source of Payment," states that "*Where Enrollee is enrolled in a Plan subject to state or federal legal requirements that prohibit a physician from billing patients for Covered Services in the event that the Payer*" (the insurer) "*fails to make such payment, the Medical Services Entity*" (doctor, hospital, or other provider) "*agrees to look solely to that Payer*" (again the insurer) "*for payment of all Covered Services delivered during the terms of the Agreement.*" Consequently, we have the AMA just accepting the fact that their membership cannot bill an enrollee for any rendered "necessary and appropriate" care that an insurer has denied in rationing health care. Furthermore, AMA offers absolutely no explanation of how these contractual restraints comply with the law or how they are to be explained to a patient. In fact, the AMA's sixty-seven page tutorial provides no discussion on the issue what-so-ever. It's a deafening silence and one that can only be by design.

This absence of any AMA-proposed counter contractual language or an explanation of how a doctor can privately contract with an enrollee to provide care that an insurer is refusing to cover is mind-blowing, particularly when the AMA, in another section of the Model Contract entitled "Medical Necessity and Due Process," states that "*Generally speaking, managed care organizations (MCOs) will pay for Covered Services that are medically necessary.*" How much clearer can it get? The AMA is acknowledging, in simple English, that there will be times when an insurer will ration care by *not* paying for what a doctor believes is the "necessary and appropriate" care an enrollee should receive. And when this occurs, the doctor may *not* contract with or bill an enrollee for this care, even if the enrollee is ready, willing and able to pay for it — *and we, the AMA, are not going to discuss these contract provisions any further.*

ERISA Preemption Manual for State Health Policy Makers

In its more than 110-page policy manual, the National-al Academy for State Health Policy devotes a mere two sentences to the state-mandated contractual provisions that bar providers from billing an enrollee. HMO licensing laws "*prohibit providers from*

53

seeking remuneration from enrollees if the plan fails to pay" (ration care) and "*States may want to require that these provider hold-harmless guarantees be part of plan-enrollee contracts in order to better defend them as insurance regulation.*" These two statements provide excellent insight into why the insurance industry and the states have been so insistent that the industry's provider contracts be treated as "*trade secrets or privileged or confidential*" commercial information (NAIC HMO Model Act).

For, while the ERISA Preemption Manual for State Health Policy Makers may advocate "*that these provider hold-harmless guarantees be part of plan-enrollee contracts in order to better defend them as insurance regulation,*" this has never happened and it most likely never will. In fact, it's counter to the very structure of managed-care health insurance. And even if one could find some way to surmount this hurdle, insurers would still have to get enrollees to <u>knowingly</u> surrender their personal and private doctor-patient relationship. Even more problematic, it would open the entire issue of rationing to public and <u>legal</u> review.

We need to understand that in order to effectively *ration* health care an insurer doesn't have to actually deny care. It only has to ensure that the provider of the care knows in advance that it can't get paid. This is the embodiment of "rationing" in the world of managed-care health insurance. After all, what hospital is going to provide care when it knows in advance that it can't get paid for costs that can easily be in the tens of thousands of dollars or more?

The bottom line is that nothing that is so central to what providers can bill and the care enrollees are allowed to receive can remain so undefined, undisclosed, and undiscussed unless the issue is being deliberately hidden. And, for those who still refuse to believe that something this large and central to our health care system is being hidden, call your insurer, your state's department of insurance, your state representative, or your U.S. congressman or senator and ask for a copy of the provider contract that defines the relationship you are allowed to have with your doctor, hospital, or any other in-network provider of health care services. *Please ask them*! I have, and I have been ignored, stonewalled, and dismissed. "The Chief of Staff for U. S. Congressman Joe Pitts went so far as to demand to know just who I thought I was to insist on pursuing this issue. He went on to tell me "*to forget*" any thought of testifying on the subject before Congressman's Pitt's Subcommittee on Health. Testimony that I was offering specifically because I had gained access to these secret contracts and wanted to share what I had learned with Congress and the American people.

(H) A Mandated Enrollee Hold Harmless Clause:

For those who believe their health insurance provides a private and personal doctor/patient relationship, you need to carefully read the states' mandated Enrollee Hold Harmless clause, which says:

Doctor agrees that in no event, including but not limited to non-payment by Insurance Company, Insurance Company's insolvency or breach of this agreement, shall Doctor, one of its subcontractors, or any of its employees or independent contractors bill, charge, collect a deposit from, seek compensation, remuneration or reimbursement from, or have any recourse against an Enrollee or persons other than the insurance company acting on behalf of Enrollee for Covered Services provided pursuant to this Agreement. This provision shall not prohibit the collection of coinsurance, co-payments or charges for Non-Covered Services. Doctor further agrees that (1) this provision shall survive the termination of this Agreement regardless of the cause giving rise to termination and shall be construed to be for the benefit of the Enrollees, and that (2) this provision supersedes any oral or written contrary agreement now existing or hereafter entered into between Doctor and Enrollees or persons acting on

their behalf. Doctor may not change, amend or waive this provision without prior written consent of the Insurance Company. Any attempt to change, amend or waive this provision are void.

In a world where no two attorneys use the same language for a contractual provision and no two states adopt the same language in a piece of legislation, the Enrollee Hold Harmless clause stands out as a clear and bold exception. Quietly imbedded in the laws and regulations of every state and mandated for incorporation in a provider contract that insurers are required to have with their in-network doctors, hospitals, and other providers of health care services, the Enrollee Hold Harmless clause has been written into millions of healthcare documents across the nation, with nothing more than the assurance that it is for the benefit of enrollees in managed-care health plans.

Much as the Trojans decorated their wooden horse to ensure that the people of Troy wouldn't look inside, the states and the insurance industry have adorned the Enrollee Hold Harmless clause with the assurance that it is for the benefit of enrollees. In essence, enrollees are told there is no reason to look inside the Clause or question the role of its language in managed-care health insurance. Just as the people of Troy stood idly by as that ancient wooden horse was pulled within their city walls, our nation has stood silent while the Enrollee Hold Harmless clause has been incorporated in every provider contract in the country. In fact, over my many years of researching the Clause, I have never found a single instance of a person or organization questioning its purpose or the reach of its language. In short, you will find not one instance of discussion or explanation of language that, on its face: 1.) Leaves no room for an enrollee to pay for "necessary and appropriate" health care an insurer denies, 2.) Bars physicians from receiving any pay whatsoever unless they accept the medical decisions of an insurer, and 3.) Irrevocably severs an enrollee's doctor-patient relationship.

Originally drafted by NAIC, the Enrollee Hold Harmless clause has become a part of the laws and regulations of every state in the country (*Study of Balanced Billing Prohibitions in Maryland*, 2002). These laws and regulations require HMOs to have a written state-approved contract with every doctor, hospital, and other provider of health care services and that these contracts must contain the Enrollee Hold Harmless clause. In fact, given the length and complexity of these mandated contracts, it is impossible to say that their reach stops at managed care. The states have allowed insurers to draft the contracts so that they cover all their many products as well as extend to all their subsidiaries, affiliates, contractors, subcontractors, and who knows how many others. In this way the insurance industry has been allowed to establish contractual control over a network of products, organizations, and providers that, literally, defies definition.

To appreciate the significance of the Enrollee Hold Harmless clause, we need only ask two of the many questions the Clause raises: 1) Can an enrollee independently contract for "necessary and appropriate" health care that an insurer refuses to approve for coverage? and 2) How does the Enrollee Hold Harmless clause affect an enrollee's doctor-patient relationship?

Enrollee Self-Payment for Denied "Necessary and Appropriate" Care:

The fact that the language of the Enrollee Hold Harmless clause leaves no room for any form of direct contracting between an in-network doctor, hospital, or other provider of health care services and an enrollee for a "Covered Service" is abundantly clear. Unfortunately, it has been my experience that this common-sense interpretation of the Clause does not apply to the insurance industry and the state departments of health and insurance. These folks stand ready and willing to assure us that the Clause does no such thing. They simply parrot that the Clause is solely limited to protecting enrollees from insurer insolvency and balance billing. In fact, I am confident the working representatives of the insurance industry and the states have repeated this explanation so often that they actually believe it's true. I heard it constantly throughout my ten years of litigating the issue. However, not once in all those years did I ever hear exactly how an enrollee could pay for a Covered Service an insurer refused to approve for coverage. Or to state it more simply, I never heard how a doctor or other provider of health care services can bill an enrollee for a Covered Service that an insurer refuses to approve. The most I have ever heard is *"We would let them pay"* or *"The enrollee is completely free to pay for a Non-Covered Service"* — statements that anyone at the top of state government or the insurance industry knows are deliberately misleading and false.

Once the Enrollee Hold Harmless clause is incorporated in a private provider contract, its interpretation is based on contract law. And, since the language is clear and there are no defined limitations or work-around provisions, the meaning of the Clause can be only exactly what the language states. Remember, a "Covered Service" is legally defined as the care that is *available* from a plan, not what an insurer elects to approve and pay for in any particular instance. Consequently, any claim by an insurer that they allow an enrollee to separately contract and pay for a "Covered Service" can only be a deliberately false statement. The Enrollee Hold Harmless clause is state-mandated language that an insurer cannot waive without legislative approval. Or to put it another way, the Enrollee Hold Harmless clause is a state-mandated provision that insurers cannot arbitrarily waive.

As to the claim that "an enrollee is completely free to pay for a 'Non-Covered Service, one really can't find a better example of the industry's willingness to mislead enrollees and the nation. Since a "Covered Service" is the care available under a plan, a "Non-Covered Service" can be only the care that is *never* available from a plan. Moreover, such "Non-Covered Services" are typically defined as elective cosmetic surgery and experimental treatments. Consequently, the Enrollee Hold Harmless clause can only be read to allow providers to bill enrollees for services associated with elective cosmetic surgery and experimental treatments. That's all. As explained to me by David Murdock, the former vice president of Legal for the Caron Foundation, *"We have tried everything, and there is just no way under the Enrollee Hold Harmless clause for an enrollee to pay for necessary health care."* Or more simply stated, there is no way for an in-network provider to get paid for the "necessary and appropriate" care your doctor has prescribed unless it agrees with what your insurer is willing to approve.

The Effect on the Doctor-Patient Relationship:

While the definition of the doctor-patient relationship has undergone significant change in recent years as legislatures and the courts have wrestled with changes brought on by the explosion in information technology, there remains broad agreement on the underlying basis for this personal and private relationship. Doctors are still expected to treat every patient with the same measure of duty, skill, and care as has always existed. Furthermore, the duty owed to the patient remains that of a fiduciary wherein the patient's interests must be paramount. Fiduciary duty comes from the Latin *fiduciarius*, meaning to hold "in trust." *Fides* means "faith," and *fiducia*, "trust." Or, as one court has stated it, *"The patient must necessarily place great reliance, faith and confidence in the professional word, advice and acts of the physician."*

Given the language in the Enrollee Hold Harmless clause, that required faith and trust simply cannot exist. After all, the only way an in-network doctor can get paid is to accept the decisions of a third-party insurer on exactly what is and is not medically "necessary and appropriate" health care. This conflict of interest not only dictates whether the doctor will be paid but: 1. Essentially assures the standard of care an enrollee is allowed to receive will be less than the highest level of available care, and 2.) Balanced against the interests of other patients and the insurer's goals for profitability. Or, to summarize this conflict of interest in an old aphorism, *"When money speaks, truth is silent."*

Most states already require physicians to disclose all material information that is required to enable a patient to make an informed decision on their health care. The California Supreme Court has even held that the doctor-patient relationship must include a physician's disclosure of all economic facts material to a patient's consent or that might affect a physician's medical judgment. Furthermore, the AMA has long advocated that physicians disclose all relevant financial interests to a patient. So how can there be any doubt that the conflict of interest created by the Enrollee Hold Harmless clause qualifies as material and relevant to a physician's judgment on "necessary and appropriate" care and an enrollee's faith and trust in a private and personal doctor-patient relationship?

In fact, the Enrollee Hold Harmless clause takes the national discussion of financial incentives to a whole new level. Up to this point, the discussion has been limited to incentives that are at the margin of the total cost of care and computed across the entire range of a doctor's many patients. Examples of these marginal incentives are where physicians are rewarded for curtailing their average cost per patient or limiting the total number of referrals to outside specialists — all justified on the basis of improving efficiency. However, the Enrollee Hold Harmless clause focuses solely on the individual enrollee and is absolute in terms of a physician's compensation. In other words, the only way an enrollee's doctor and other in-network providers can get paid is to accept the medical decisions of a third-party insurer that employs rationing to reduce the cost of care.

Consider for a moment how a hospital might react if an attending physician insisted on prescribing care that both knew could not be billed. Regardless of whether the doctor is an independent practitioner or an employee of the hospital, he or she would be threatening the hospital with tens of thousands of dollars in unpaid costs and subjecting themselves to some form of significant retribution.

What makes all this even worse is that by signing a provider contract with its Enrollee Hold Harmless clause, an enrollee's doctor accepts a confidentiality provision that bars any disclosure of the Clause. Consequently, a doctor can be rightly accused of direct participation in a scheme to hide both the conflict of interest created by the Clause and the liability attached to it. How can a doctor argue that he remains an unbiased advocate for a patient's care when the only way he or she can get paid is to accept a third party's medical decision on "necessary and appropriate" health care? Furthermore, how can a physician argue that he doesn't understand the severity of the restriction when physicians can be shown to struggle with this reality every day of their practice?

(I) Your Right to Coverage When Insurers Say "No":

As Justice Souter so aptly wrote in Pegram v. Herdrich, the *"inducement to ration care is the very point of any HMO scheme."* However, the inducement to ration care is a far cry from the actual authority to ration care under U. S. law. The rationing of health care, by its very nature, requires the power to overrule the medical judgment of a properly licensed attending physician — a physician who has been given the sole authority to prescribe medically "necessary and appropriate" health care. In fact, this authority is so firmly embedded in state law that it cannot be changed any more than the laws limiting specific decision-making to properly licensed engineers, attorneys, or CPAs. Furthermore, so long as there is an offer to pay for this lawfully prescribed "necessary and appropriate" health care, a licensed hospital has to agree to provide it if it's within their capability. That is the law in every state of the country. In essence, so long as the care is prescribed by your doctor and there is <u>some</u> offer to pay for it, a hospital must agree to supply it or find another hospital that can. This is the well-established law in the United States that managed-care and the states have had to overcome in order to ration health care. It's also a body of law that gives your managed-care insurer a very real Achilles heel.

In order to both avoid a charge of practicing medicine and allow insurers to overrule the lawful decision of an attending physician (your doctor), the managed-care insurance industry and the states have created provider contracts that deprive every in-network physician, hospital or other in-network provider of health care services of all compensation unless they accept an insurer's authority to ration care. The obvious line of thought being that if providers know they can't get paid, they will be forced to accept the insurer's decisions on rationing health care. It's an extremely effective design. Unfortunately for the insurance industry, it's also a design with a huge Achilles heel. It's what I describe as the *back door* to care and coverage.

Because the insurance industry's contractual approach to rationing fails to change the law in any way, the attending physician (your doctor) is still the only one authorized to determine medically "necessary and appropriate" health care. Consequently: 1.) Hospitals are required to provide the prescribed care as long as there is <u>an</u> offer to pay, 2.) Your offer to pay must be accepted as a matter of law, and 3.) The fact that the hospital or other provider of health care service has secretly and voluntarily surrendered their right to bill you is not your concern. Simply stated, you have every right to demand the care prescribed by your doctor, demand your right to pay for it, sign any promise to pay that is requested and then refuse the bill as a legally unenforceable debt. It's simply your right under the law and the Achilles heel that their approach to rationing creates. Furthermore, you have a clear and well held right to this *back door* approach as you are doing nothing more than collecting the *coverage* your plan has been structured to provide, regardless of all the huffing and puffing by your insurer or provider. Remember, as an enrollee you have never signed anything and never agreed to the insurer's terms and conditions. Furthermore, any pursuit of payment by a provider or insurer would force the disclosure of these provider contracts along with their Enrollee Hold Harmless clause — something neither the insurance industry nor the states can afford to accept. In total, **it's a truth about provider contracts and the law that the managed-care insurance industry and the states need to keep hidden!**

Rather than appeal an insurer's decision to deny coverage and provide the time the insurer needs to twist the arm of the attending physician, enrollees have every right to simply execute the terms of the insurer's provider contract and the law. After all, it's no coincidence that an insurer's appeal process is designed to take considerable time. It takes time to twist the arm of a conscientious doctor. The appeal process provides that necessary time. It also assures the insurer of success because time brings change in a patient's condition that can only serve to blur the entire issue of appropriate care and coverage as well as eliminate any insurer liability. In the case of my former wife, our insurer was so confident in their ability to change our doctor's decision on the care Sandy needed that they actually told me what her doctor would decide before they got her to change her mind, i.e., before Sandy's doctor agreed to accept the insurer's decision on the care Sandy would be allowed to receive.

The bottom line is that the provider contracts that all in-network providers are required to sign, including your doctor, guarantee an enrollee's right to the care prescribed by their doctor, regardless of what an insurer decides on care and coverage. Insurers and the states just don't want us to know it.

(J) Their Fraudulent Bills:

Of all the fraud and misrepresentation in managed-care health insurance, fraudulent billing is the most egregious. However, as bad as it is, it offers the nation a "silver bullet" that can force reform of our national health care system. This is not so much because the fraud allows attorneys to pursue reform through the courts, but because it allows individual enrollees to reject most of what hospitals have been billing enrollees for more than twenty years. It's a large part of the "Too Big to Be Legal" title for the book.

Because this fraudulent billing is covered in great detail in a later section of the book, I will limit my comments here so as not to repeat myself. For now I will just say that one needs only to apply the language of the Enrollee Hold Harmless clause to a typical hospital bill to begin to get a feel for the breadth and depth of the fraudulent billing that the health care industry has concocted to line their pockets and fleece unsuspecting enrollees.

We can begin with a simple example involving something we all understand. Let's say we go shopping for the family's weekly groceries and the clerk at the register merely presents us with a total owed. There is no printed list of what we have in our cart or the price of the items and no indication of whether we are being charged the regular price for the turkey or the sale price that brought us into the store. We are given nothing that would allow us to compare the prices we are being charged with what we have in our shopping cart and what we should be paying. This is the exact situation an enrollee faces following a stay in a hospital.

Quoting from a hospital bill I recently received: **Total Charges:** $40,713.24; **Insurance Payments to Date:** $3,146.46; **Adjustments to Date:** $36,621.71; **Your Responsibility:** $945.07. That was the complete explanation of what they clearly wanted me to pay. It was also the total explanation of what I owed after review by, I would hope, three separate insurance plans that my wife and I are fortunate enough to have. Furthermore, when I questioned this lack of detailed accounting, I was assured it was because enrollees do not want to be bothered with all the detailed information that necessarily goes into computing a lengthy hospital bill. However, just for fun, let's apply the Enrollee Hold Harmless clause to the unwanted, bothersome details in my hospital bill. Let's compare my bill with what the hospital, or any other billing entity, would have to provide to make their bill legally enforceable.

As a matter of well-established law, the hospital has to provide me with a list of not only the services I received, but the price it is charging for each one of them. However, we are not talking about the prices a hospital lists in what they refer to as their published Chargemaster. We are talking about the discounted prices that my insurance company has negotiated with the hospital for the befit of all the enrollees in my managed-care health plan. More specifically, we are talking about the prices in the hospital's provider contract. Unfortunately for everyone, this is a secret contract that specifically bars <u>any</u> disclosure of these discounted prices. Furthermore, since, at least in my case, I have three separate plans, just which secret price list is appropriate? I have to assume that all three apply. And then there is the problem that the hospital cannot bill me for any service (individual charge) that any one of my three plans has denied for coverage or payment, i.e., the Enrollee Hold Harmless clause. And, believe me, I have only begun to touch the complexity of what my hospital needs to provide to justify its bill. So why trouble me with all those "unwanted" and annoying details that limit what they can bill me? Why limit what they can justifiably bill when they can simply compute their own **"Pay This Amount"** and move it to collection if I fail to pay?

For those lawyers who would argue that this doesn't necessarily constitute intentional fraud, please consider the following. I received two separate but similar bills from two different hospitals for hospitalization in the past year. In each case I spoke with a supervisor and explained that, given the law and the contracts they have signed, this was not my bill but theirs, and the bill was, at best, overstated. The response of the two supervisors was almost identical and can be characterized as, "Oh, we have made a mistake. Don't do anything. We will take care of it." I haven't heard a word from either of them since.

One particularly amazing part of this fraud that I must mention here is that the wording of the Enrollee Hold Harmless clause in Pennsylvania law appears to contractually bar hospitals and all other in-network providers from billing an enrollee for a "deductible" or any costs in excess of a defined "cap" on coverage. In other words, even if an enrollee's plan calls for the enrollee to pay a deductible or is subject to a cap on coverage, there is no provision in Pennsylvania law that I am aware of that entitles an in-network provider to bill an enrollee for these unpaid amounts.

An insurer simply denies payment based on what they see as the limits in a specific plan, just as they do when they deny payment based on their determination of "necessary and appropriate" care. Consequently, providers can only see an insurer's failure to pay as it would any other failure to pay that is subject to the Enrollee Hold Harmless clause and <u>one that they cannot bill to an enrollee</u>.

Before we all jump to the defense of the poor suffering hospitals, let's consider this: "*Thousands of hospitals have morphed into high-profit, high-profile businesses . . . that buy more equipment, hire more people, offer more services, buy rival hospitals and then raise executive salaries because their operations have gotten so much larger. It's a uniquely American gold rush*" (Steven Brill, "Why Medical Bills Are Killing Us," *Time* magazine, March 4, 2013).

(K) The Unholy Alliance with States:

Managed-care health insurance is supposed to function pretty much like our justice system. Where the justice system promises us our own attorney and a fair and impartial judiciary, managed care promises us our own doctor and a fair and impartial state department of insurance. Remember, the states are charged with overseeing the "business" of insurance and review and approve every plan insurers market as well as scrutinize the marketing and sales practices of these plans. That is to say, the states are responsible for maintaining a fair and stable insurance marketplace that benefits the public. So it's entirely reasonable for enrollees to look to the departments of insurance and health, or the equivalent in a state, when an insurer fails to deliver on the coverage promised by a managed-care health plan. In fact, the states actively encourage such requests for help in order to keep complaints away from the courts. And, until I got well into researching the material for this second book, I would have agreed that a state department of insurance is the logical place to look for help in a dispute with an insurance company. I really wanted to believe that my state put the interests of the individual enrollee ahead of those of an insurance industry. Unfortunately, I once again could not have been more wrong.

As stated earlier, for the first forty years of its existence, managed-care health insurance simply provided *"whatever procedures"* an enrollee's doctor *"chose to order and perform"* ("Decreasing Variation in Medical Necessity Decision Making," Center for Health Policy Making, Stanford University, 1999). During that time the term *medical necessity* was called an *"innocuous placeholder"* that allowed physicians to make judgments on care and coverage that went largely *"unchallenged"* (again from the 1999 Stanford University Report). After all, the early insurers were focused only on getting in-network doctors and hospitals paid.

Passage of the 1973 HMO Act changed the landscape of health care in the United States by putting the federal government squarely behind the growth of employer-supplied managed-care health insurance. Consequently, by the early 1990s, HMOs dominated the American health care market. Unfortunately, this explosive growth put the health care market in crisis. The nation experienced a raft of HMO insolvencies, federal bankruptcy courts threatened the states' authority to regulate insurance, there was a growing HMO backlash for excessive denials of care and coverage, and insurers were under increasing pressure to cut the cost of health care. Something had to be done. That something can best be summed up as the restructuring of provider contracts that contained NAIC's Enrollee Hold Harmless clause, all cloaked in the promise to provide enrollees greater protection from the issues that HMOs had created.

By mandating the inclusion of the NAIC's Enrollee Hold Harmless clause in newly constructed provider contracts, the states: 1.) Gave insurers permission to contractually grant themselves the "discretion" to determine "necessary and appropriate" care for insurance purposes (the rationing of health care) rather than the heretofore practice of simply making their own *medical* determination of "necessary and appropriate" care, 2.) Resolved the federal bankruptcy issue, and 3.) Gave the public the perception of a more regulated and responsible insurance industry.

Prior to these changes, managed-care insurers had learned *"through harsh experience with the courts that there was little point in continuing to rely on vague language they know will be construed against them*" ("The Futility of Medical Necessity," E. Haavi Morreim, 2001). However, when the debate is "*over the discretion to construe or interpret contract terms, there is very little discussion about the meaning of medical necessity*" ("The Debate Over Medical Necessity," Foundation for the Advancement of Innovative Medicine, 2001). In other words, by restructuring their provider contracts to contractually give themselves the *discretion* to determine "necessary and appropriate" care and then use the Enrollee Hold Harmless clause to force doctors to agree with their decisions, insurers effectively eliminated their liability for denying coverage and rationing health care. "*The upshot is that when discretion of the insurer is protected by contract, the use of that discretion to interpret contract terms, like medical necessity, cannot be challenged unless the patient can prove that the discretion was used capriciously or arbitrarily*" ("The Debate Over Medical Necessity in Case Law," Foundation for the Advancement of Innovative Medicine, 1998).

My point here is that the states have been, and continue to be, a full and active participant in defending managed care's ability to deny coverage and ration health care on the basis of an insurer's determination of "necessary and appropriate" care. It's a point that is easy to prove. All one needs to do is to ask their state department of insurance, or its equivalent, how an enrollee's in-network doctor can contract, render, and bill a Covered Service their insurer refuses to approve and cover as "necessary and appropriate" health care. Ask, and then watch the dance that follows. I guarantee it will be entertaining. It will also provide all the proof one needs of the unholy alliance between the state and the managed-care insurance industry — an alliance where the interests of the individual enrollee are secondary to what are viewed as the larger needs of the managed-care insurance industry and government.

For those who might still believe the states could never be complicit in usurping a doctor's authority to determine medically "necessary and appropriate" health care, look at states like Pennsylvania and New York, which have incorporated provisions in their laws that grant insurers the authority to determine "necessary and appropriate" care while maintaining other provisions that limit this authority to properly licensed attending physicians. These states have made no effort to separate these obviously conflicting provisions in their laws or to separate the role of the insurer from the role of the attending physician in determining the care a patient is allowed to receive. Instead, the states have promoted a steady blurring of the line between the authority of insurers to make insurance decisions from the authority of attending physicians to make medical decisions. It's a blurring of the line that is so obvious that it would be ludicrous to claim the states are unaware of the consequences of their actions. Furthermore, it's a shift in policy that, initially, *"neither consumers nor their physicians were fully aware of"* (Monica Miller, Stanford University Report, 1999).

To be fair to the states, they didn't create this mess. In fact, one can reasonably argue that the states have done no more than deal with what the federal government handed them. When Congress passed the 1973 HMO Act, they put the full weight of the federal government behind the growth of employer-supplied managed-care health insurance. As I mentioned earlier, this created a significant regulatory problem for the states because a managed-care health plan is not insurance. Therefore, it could be easily viewed as an area for federal oversight. Nowhere was this more evident than in the area of bankruptcy. And, since the protection offered by federal bankruptcy laws was attractive to troubled HMOs, the states needed a solution that barred insolvent HMOs from accessing the protection offered by federal bankruptcy proceedings, i.e., the Enrollee Hold Harmless clause. The question then becomes whether states could have limited the reach of the Clause and still retained their authority to regulate insurance. Or, could the states have constructed the Clause so that an individual enrollee could pay for care if coverage was denied? The answer to both questions in this non-attorney's opinion is a big fat "no."

In order to retain their authority to regulate managed-care health insurance, the states had to be able to regulate insurance in all its phases of operation. This obviously had to include the authority to resolve the issue of bankruptcy. In other words, the states had to be able to provide the services and protections of federal bankruptcy proceedings, but to do so outside the domain of the federal courts. Unfortunately, the only way to do that was to eliminate the issues that a failing insurer could properly plead to a federal bankruptcy court. In essence, the states needed providers to have formally accepted: 1.) zero payment as payment in full when an insurer fails to pay for services rendered to an enrollee, and 2.) the surrender of any and all right to bill an enrollee in such instances. Anything less would have created a hole big enough for a sharp attorney from an insurance company to drive a truck through.

The result is that the "unholy alliance" between the states and the managed-care insurance industry comes from their need to defend the Enrollee Hold Harmless clause and what the Clause does for each of them. In the case of the states, they get to support the insurance that Congress has established as the model for the country as well as retain their authority to regulate the business of health insurance. In the case of the managed-care insurance industry, they get the power to enforce their rationing by requiring providers to accept zero payment unless they accept the insurer's decisions on the coverage. And they both get to claim, or at least rationalize, that they are doing what the country needs to reduce the cost of health care — all for the greater good.

A Perfect Example:

In 2004 the fact that health insurance companies in Pennsylvania were refusing to approve hospitalization for drug and alcohol addiction as required by Pennsylvania law became so obvious that the state's insurance commissioner was forced to clarify who could determine whether an enrollee needed such care. And, because the applicable legislation (Pennsylvania Act 106, 40 P.S. §§ 908-1-908-8) specifically assigned that authority to a "licensed physician or licensed psychologist," the commissioner's statement (Notice 2003-06, 33 Pa. Bull. 4041-42, August 9, 2003) said the same thing. The Insurance Federation of Pennsylvania, along with

The Managed Care Association of Pennsylvania, Aetna, Blue Cross, and others immediately filed suit against the Insurance Department in the Commonwealth Court of Pennsylvania. They claimed that the Notice reversed fourteen years of state policy where insurers were both authorized and encouraged to have the final say on what enrollees could *receive* as "necessary and appropriate" care.

What makes this case so unique is that both parties to the suit agreed the issue was purely one of law and unique to the care and treatment of enrollees suffering from drug and alcohol dependency. In other words, the arguments on both sides acknowledged that the legislature had authorized and encouraged insurers to have the final say on the care enrollees could receive. Therefore, they agreed that the issue before the court was solely one of whether the legislature had created an exception for enrollees suffering from drug and alcohol addiction.

This issue was "so important" to the state that a final decision in the case didn't come until May 27, 2009, a full six years after the issues surfaced. The Pennsylvania Supreme Court ruled that: 1.) The intent of the legislature is clear in that Act 106 specifically states that a "licensed physician or licensed psychologist" is to determine the care needed for drug and alcohol addiction, 2.) The Insurance Department's 2003 Notice was simply *"a statement of policy, without binding effect"* and *"does not establish a binding norm,"* and 3.) Insurer's right to have the final say in the care enrollees can receive in all other instances has *"been properly recognized by the Commonwealth Court."*

Not once in the six years of litigating the case did either side ever question the right of an insurer to overrule an enrollee's doctor or psychologist when determining the care an enrollee <u>can receive</u>. Not once did the best minds in the insurance industry, the state's Department of Insurance, the Office of the Attorney General, and both the Commonwealth Court and the Pennsylvania Supreme Court do anything that explained the authority under which the state or a managed-care insurance company can overrule an individual's doctor or psychologist on the care an enrollee *can receive*. Not once in six years of litigation did these great minds ever raise the issue that cost my wife, Sandy, her life, i.e., the decision of her insurer to deny the care her doctor certified as absolutely necessary. Instead, the participants in this case, including the Pennsylvania Supreme Court, openly agreed that prior to 2003, the insurance companies in Pennsylvania were *encouraged* to overrule attending physicians in determining needed care, and the Department's 2003 Notice is *"merely an announcement to the public of the policy which the agency hopes to implement in future rulemaking or adjudications"* in the narrow area of drug and alcohol addiction — something it has never done.

The bottom line is that these six years of litigation provide an unusually open and explicit example of how deeply the states are involved in maintaining the insurance industry's authority to have the final say on the care an enrollee is *allowed to receive*. After all, it took six years to rule that the language in Act 106 specifically states that the *"authority"* to determine care and to refer an enrollee for treatment rests with a *"licensed physician or licensed psychologist,"* six years to ensure that the final ruling *"does not establish a binding norm"* on the industry, and six years to ensure that the insurance industry's authority to overrule an enrollee's doctor for the purpose of rationing "necessary and appropriate" health care remains unchanged.

FIVE

*"Obamacare lets the bear
into the room:"*
Noted Wilmington Attorney

Why Obamacare Changes Everything

Throughout the writing of this book, all I heard from the various news sources were reports on how my Republican Party, particularly conservatives, were obsessed with repealing Obamacare. Led by Heritage Action of The Heritage Foundation, conservatives described themselves as hell-bent on doing whatever it took to block the implementation of Obamacare. Or, stating it more specifically, they claimed to be willing to do whatever it would take to kill the implementation of the individual mandate in Obamacare.

Their Earlier Support for a Mandate:

The surprising part of all this is that The Heritage Foundation was one of the first, if not the first, to propose an individual mandate. In a brief written by Stuart Butler of The Heritage Foundation in 1998 entitled "Assuring Affordable Health Care for All Americans," Heritage laid out a vision for health care reform that would *"mandate all households to obtain adequate insurance."* The brief went on to describe the mandate as the way to resolve the *"free rider"* problem in the existing health care system. The *"free riders"* were described as individuals without insurance who force the public to pay for their care in hospital emergency rooms. This Heritage Foundation brief further stated that if an individual *"has spent his money on other things rather than insurance, we may be angry but we will not deny him services, even if that means more prudent citizens end up paying the tab."* And a mandate on households would force *"those with adequate means to obtain insurance protection, which would end the problem of middle-class free riders on society's sense of obligation"* (Stuart Butler).

However, this was not the first time the Republican Party had provided support for an individual mandate. Mark Pauly, Senior Professor of Health Care Management at the University of Pennsylvania, along with a number of other leaders in health care, included it in a proposal they submitted to President George H. W. Bush in 1991. The individual mandate was at the *"heart"* of this proposal (Professor Pauly, Washington Post, Ezra Klein Editorial, January 1, 2011). While Professor Pauly wasn't a member of the Bush Administration, he was teamed with a number of health care professionals to develop a conservative proposal to serve as an alternative to the universal payer model that was being advocated by leading Democrats. This conservative proposal was published in *Health Affairs* in 1991. However, it was declared dead on arrival by the Democrats.

Not to be so easily dissuaded, key conservatives and Republicans in Congress throughout 1992 and 1993 continued to include the mandate in a number of alternative proposals to what was being proposed by the Clinton administration, i.e., Hillarycare. One such bill was the "Health Equity and Access Reform Today Act," introduced in the Senate in 1993. It was co-sponsored by staunch conservative Senators Chuck Grassley and Orrin Hatch and nearly half the Republicans in the U. S. Senate. Referred to as the "Heart Act," it called for federal vouchers to help low-income individuals buy health insurance and <u>a mandate that all Americans obtain adequate health insurance</u>. Newt Gingrich, the Republican minority leader in the House, openly supported the mandate. In fact he continued to support the idea until as late as May 2011. So what changed? What caused Republicans and conservatives, who were once so willing to accept an individual mandate that all Americans have adequate health insurance, to view the mandate in Obamacare as anathema to acceptable health care reform?

In all fairness to Heritage, conservatives, and Republicans, their position has been quite consistent if we look closely at what they were proposing. On the other hand, I will argue that a close look at what they were proposing will also demonstrate their willingness to ignore the constitutional rights of the individual enrollee in managed-care health insurance in order to avoid subjecting the managed-care insurance industry to a constitutional challenge they cannot win. And, I am not talking about whether the individual mandate is constitutional. The U. S. Supreme Court settled that issue. So, for the moment, let's put the constitutional issue aside. Let's concern ourselves only with what Heritage, conservatives, and my Republican Party leadership have been proposing for the past twenty-some years.

Fortunately, we have been given a great deal of help because The Heritage Foundation, Republicans and conservatives have been forced to respond to fierce criticism from the left and the press for what many see as a stark reversal in their position on an individual mandate. Furthermore, this criticism has specifically cited Heritage as once being the leading advocate for an individual mandate. In responding to this criticism, Stuart Butler of The Heritage Foundation wrote an op-ed in *USA Today* describing as a myth the idea that Heritage had invented the individual mandate. He wrote that "*I headed Heritage's health work for thirty years. Make no mistake: Heritage and I actively oppose the individual mandate.*" Butler described Heritage's "supposed" support for a mandate as purely a "*technical matter*" that sought to draw a contrast with President Clinton's Hillarycare.

Butler went on to write, "*The confusion arises from the fact that twenty years ago, I held the view that as a technical matter, some form of requirement to purchase insurance was needed in the near-*

universal insurance market to avoid massive instability through adverse selection (insurers avoiding bad risks and healthy people declining coverage). At that time, President Clinton was proposing a universal health care plan, and Heritage and I devised a viable alternative."

"My view was shared at the time by many conservative experts, including American Enterprise Institute (AEI) scholars, as well as most non-conservative analysts. Even libertarian-conservative icon Milton Friedman, in a 1991 Wall Street Journal *article, advocated replacing Medicare and Medicaid with a requirement that every U. S. family unit have a major medical insurance policy."*

As a Republican, a conservative, and one who is willing to take Stuart Butler at his word, I'll accept that Heritage didn't "<u>invent</u>" the idea of an individual mandate. And I am more than willing to accept his explanation that Heritage's proposal for an individual mandate was merely a "<u>technical alternative</u>" to Hillarycare and one that was "<u>shared at the time by many conservative experts</u>." However, how can something that was so openly supported by Heritage and leading conservatives for twenty years and was in Butler's own words "an acceptable alternative" now be so damaging and unacceptable that it is worth shutting down the government and threatening the faith and credit of the nation? How can my Republican party ask me and the rest of the country to believe that these draconian measures can be explained by the fact that we have simply changed our mind on something we supported for twenty-some years? *"The way it was viewed by the Congressional Budget Office in 1994,"* the mandate *"was, effectively, a tax . . . so I've been surprised by the argument"* (Professor Pauly, Washington Post, Ezra Klein Editorial, January 1, 2011).

No Clear Reason for the Change:

Once again trying to be fair to Heritage, conservatives, and my Republican Party, and using their own words, I have to admit that there is a definable difference between what they supported for twenty-some years and the individual mandate in Obamacare. Where

Heritage, conservatives, and my Republican Party have advocated for a mandate in the form of a tax credit, Obamacare makes the mandate a requirement in federal law rather than a tax advantage or voucher for purchasing acceptable health insurance. In other words, rather than establishing a tax advantage or voucher system to encourage compliance with an individual mandate, Obamacare makes the mandate an actual requirement in federal law and levies a tax penalty on all those who fail to comply. This may be a small distinction to the vast majority of us and the press, but I assure you it is no small distinction to Heritage and other conservative and Republican experts on health insurance. However, it was a small enough distinction for the U.S. Supreme Court to disappoint Heritage, conservatives and Republicans and rule that the mandate in Obamacare is, in fact, constitutional.

In attempting to explain Heritage's opposition to Obamacare, Stuart Butler's op-ed in *USA Today* provided four reasons why he and Heritage are currently so opposed to the mandate in Obamacare: 1.) It is no longer necessary, 2.) Improving stability in the voluntary insurance market makes it no longer necessary, 3.) Obamacare forces individuals to purchase comprehensive coverage rather than catastrophic coverage, and 4.) Obama's mandate is unconstitutional.

Excuse me, I may not be an attorney or a health care expert, but I can certainly recognize a manufactured explanation when I see one. No one is going to convince me that reasons one, two, and three are anything but a smokescreen for reason number four. And no one is going to convince me that something that Heritage, leading conservatives and my Republican Party supported for twenty-some years is so damningly unconstitutional. Think what you may, but these are reasonable and very knowledgeable people and no reasonable and knowledgeable people are going support something so damningly unconstitutional for twenty-odd years, particularly when these people are committed to protecting our constitutional rights. Even more obvious is that no reasonable and knowledgeable people are going to shut down the government and threaten to destroy the faith and credit of the country over an issue that their twenty years of support and a review by the Supreme Court have confirmed is constitutional. There has to be something else, something we are missing, some other issue that leading conservatives have with the mandate in Obamacare.

Again being fair to Stuart Butler and Heritage in attempting to understand Mr. Butler's explanation of why he, Heritage, other conservatives and my Republican Party are so opposed to Obamacare, I hope we can agree that the core of their objections can't be Mr. Butler's reasons one, two, or three. They simply aren't material enough to justify shutting down the government and threatening the faith and credit of the nation. Furthermore, I have to believe that Mr. Butler and Heritage are honest and responsible people. So Mr. Butler's four reasons can't be deliberately false. That leaves only the constitutional issue (reason four) to justify such blatant extremism. However, the Supreme Court has already ruled that the mandate in Obamacare is constitutional. And, yet, Heritage, conservatives and the Republican Party are more determined than ever to kill Obamacare — to kill a mandate that is expected to deliver forty million new customers to the private insurance industry that Heritage and the Republican Party actively support. So, what are we missing? Why are these reasonable and knowledgeable people so afraid of Obamacare? Why are Mr. Butler, Heritage, conservatives and the Republican Party so obsessed with repealing Obamacare and its individual mandate?

The Real Issue Behind Efforts to Kill Obamacare:

Mr. Butler's reason four says that the mandate in Obamacare is unconstitutional. But I submit that this is not how this statement should be read. That's what we're missing. By making the mandate a requirement in federal law, the issue of constitutionality goes well beyond the mandate itself. It attaches to everything the mandate requires Americans to purchase — the entire makeup of the managed-care insurance product that Americans must buy, i.e., managed-care health insurance with all its hidden policies, practices, and rationing. That is because there can be no separation between the mandate and what it requires of the American people. In essence, it isn't the mandate that concerns Mr. Butler, Heritage, conservatives and the Republican Party; it's the constitutionality of the policies, practices, and rationing in managed-care health insurance that the Obamacare mandate exposes to federal law — an exposure they have successfully avoided under state law. To quote Edward J. Feulner, president of The Heritage Foundation in a letter to me dated May 31, 2013, *"Much of health insurance law and regulation remains within the jurisdiction of the states. I hasten to add, under our federal system, that is where it should remain"* (See Appendix #4).

The individual mandate in Obamacare irrevocably changes what Mr. Feulner and Heritage argue *"should remain"* in state law and opens managed-care health insurance and their plans to the full range of federal requirements dealing with disclosure, process, contract, liberty, and privacy — issues that heretofore were solely subject to state law in what I have described above as an "The Unholy Alliance with the States."

Prior to Obamacare, the insurance industry's alliance with the states had the effect of insulating insurers from federal law. Insurers were essentially free to overrule attending physicians in rationing "necessary and appropriate" health care while ignoring the constitutional rights of enrollees to disclosure, process, contract, liberty, and privacy in accessing health care. As a senior attorney with one of the nation's largest companies put it, the Obamacare mandate *"lets the bear into the room."* In other words, the Obamacare mandate subjects the policies, practices, and rationing embodied in managed-care health insurance to federal law and it's clear and well founded constitutional protections. It's an exposure I would have hoped Heritage, Conservatives and my Republican Party would have welcomed.

Please understand that this is not conjecture on my part, because I have discussed these conclusions with leaders in my party like the president of The Heritage Foundation, David Boaz of the Cato Institute, Clark Neely, a constitutional attorney with the Institute for Justice, U. S. Congressman Joe Pitts, the chair of the U. S. House Subcommittee on Health, State Senator Dominic Pileggi, the Republican leader of the Pennsylvania Senate and many more. Not one of these individuals has offered an alternative explanation. To quote Congressman Pitts, "*Why should I care if I can't pay for my own health care?*" And to quote his angry chief of staff, "*Who do you think you are*" and "*You can forget about being allowed to testify*" on this issue.

If I have learned anything in my seventy-six years, it's that reasonable and knowledgeable people don't act irresponsibly. The constitutionality of the Obamacare mandate is an already settled issue that pales in comparison to the constitutionality of the policies and practices that the managed-care insurance industry use to ration health care. To again quote U. S. Supreme Court Justice David Souter in the unanimous decision in Pegram v. Herdrich, "*Inducement to ration care is the very point of any H.M.O. scheme*" and "*No H.M.O organization could survive without some incentive connecting physician reward with treatment rationing.*" Please remember that whether it's an HMO, PPO, or any other acronym a managed-care insurer elects to use, it's all the same in form, function, and state-approved provider contracts. In essence, it's a single managed-care system specifically designed to ration health care in ways enrollees are not permitted to see. Consequently, Obamacare creates an exposure to federal law that the states and the insurance industry have avoided for more than twenty years — an exposure capable of creating real fear in those who see private insurance with hidden rationing as an acceptable solution to the nation's unacceptably high cost of health care.

Once again, I say that reasonable and knowledgeable people always have a good reason for their actions. In this case, one only has to recognize that Obamacare isn't the issue. The real issue for Stuart Butler, The Heritage Foundation, leading conservatives, and my Republican Party are the policies, practices, and rationing embodied in managed-care health insurance that cannot survive exposure to federal law.

SIX

....

> *"I believe there are more instances
> of the abridgment of the freedom of
> the people by gradual and silent en-
> croachments of those in power than
> in violent and sudden usurpations:"*
> James Madison

Blatantly Unconstitutional

Perhaps the best way to demonstrate why Stuart Butler, The Heritage Foundation, conservatives and Republican Party are so fearful of the individual mandate in Obamacare is to provide an analogy that we can all relate to.

States have long required the operators of motor vehicles to purchase automobile insurance before receiving a driver's license. It's a well-accepted practice in every state in the country. Furthermore, it's one I hope we can all agree is constitutional. However, what would happen if the only available automobile insurance contains a state-approved provision that strips policyholders of the right to an attorney in any dispute over the insurer's failure to pay a claim?

Viewed on its own, a state requirement that drivers obtain adequate automobile insurance is both reasonable and constitutional. Furthermore, an insurance policy limitation on representation would be simply a contractual agreement between two consenting private parties. However, once the insurance becomes the only available insurance that meets a state's requirement for appropriate insurance, the two provisions can no longer be viewed separately, and the question of constitutionality attaches to the two provisions collectively. What was a reasonable and constitutional requirement that all motor vehicle operators possess acceptable automobile insurance becomes a state mandate that all licensed motor vehicle operators surrender their right to representation in any dispute with the state's only approved form of automobile insurance.

This is the very problem that Obamacare creates for Heritage, conservatives and the Republican Party as well as the managed-care insurance industry. By making the individual mandate in Obamacare a requirement in law rather than a preferential tax rate, voucher, or government payment for the purchase of insurance, Obamacare attaches the entire structure of managed-care health insurance to the question of constitutionality and a host of other federal requirements — all outside the limits created by ERISA. After all, just as in our automobile insurance example, managed-care health insurance is effectively the only available insurance in the market. This is due, in large part, to the federal government's direct support of employer-supplied managed-care health insurance following passage of the 1973 HMO Act. In short, Congress has both intended and succeeded in effectively making managed-care health insurance the only form of health insurance that is available in the U. S. market.

So when I say Obamacare is blatantly unconstitutional, I am not referring to the Obamacare mandate itself. That question has been well settled by the recent Supreme Court decision. I am referring to the constitutionality of the Obamacare mandate when attached to state-structured managed-care health insurance that individuals must acquire.

However, since this involves two separate areas of law, one federal and one state, the issue of constitutionality must attach to one more than the other. In fact, this is at the heart of why Stuart Butler, Heritage, conservatives, and the Republican Party are so obsessively opposed to Obamacare.

Article VI, Section 2 of the U. S. Constitution states that

the "*Constitution and the laws of the United States . . . shall be the supreme law of the land . . . anything in the Constitution or laws of any State to the contrary notwithstanding*." Commonly referred to as the Supremacy Clause, this provision in the U. S. Constitution means that any federal law, even a regulation written by a federal agency, trumps any conflicting state law. Consequently, since the Obamacare mandate is both constitutional and supreme in law, the issue of constitutionality attaches to the states' structure for managed-care health insurance and their scheme for rationing health care. In short, the issue becomes the constitutionality of managed-care itself, along with its deliberately hidden system for rationing health care.

Not being an attorney and certainly having no credible claim to being a constitutional scholar, I will readily agree that the range of issues raised by the Supremacy Clause go well beyond my capability and the scope of this book. However, the analysis here appears very straightforward.

Two issues arise when a state law or policy is in apparent conflict with federal law and the Constitution's Supremacy Clause. The first is whether the congressional action falls within the powers the U. S. Constitution grants to Congress. The second is whether Congress intended its policy to supersede state policy. In this particular case, both answers appear readily available and virtually a slam-dunk in law.

In answer to the first question, Congress passed the 1973 HMO Act more than forty years ago, and no one has raised a question of its constitutionality. So I sincerely hope we can begin by accepting, as fact, that the 1973 HMO Act is both constitutional and fully within the powers granted to Congress under the U. S. Constitution. In answer to the second question, Congress clearly intended its policy on employer-supplied managed-care health insurance to be the law of the land as of 1973. This is further evidenced by Congress' passage of ERISA in 1979 which, in part, severely limits state authority in the area of employer-supplied managed-care health insurance. And, since the states didn't create their requirements for state-approved provider contracts with an Enrollee Hold Harmless clause until twenty years later, these state requirements are subject to the earlier federal policy and law on employer-supplied managed-care health insurance — insurance that applies to roughly eighty percent of Americans and more than ninety-five percent of the existing health care insurance market.

The inescapable conclusion is that unless Mr. Butler, Heritage, conservative and the Republican Party, along with the insurance industry, can find some way to make the states' policy for rationing "supreme," they and the states face exposure to the full range of federal law. In particular they face a constitutional review of the severing of an enrollee's doctor-patient relationship through hidden contractual provisions that <u>infringe an enrollee's right to contract, process, liberty, and privacy in accessing needed health care</u>.

Viewed solely as policies and practices subject to state law, as Edwin Feulner of The Heritage Foundation argues ("*Much of health insurance law and regulation remains within the jurisdiction of the states,[and] that is where it should remain*") there would be little reason to expect any significant judicial review of what is a state-supported and hidden system for rationing health care. However, once these hidden provisions and practices are subject to the bright light of federal oversight, the managed-care insurance industry and their supporters have no place to hide. The policies and practices that have been so easily hidden from enrollees and the general public under state law are in hard documents that are all-to readily available to any federal court and litigating attorney.

The bottom line is that the individual mandate in Obamacare will inevitably force the states and the insurance industry to defend their right to secretly sever an enrollee's doctor-patient relationship as well as an enrollee's right to access "necessary and appropriate" health care at their own expense. Even worse, the mandate will force this defense into a federal court system that has already ruled that a local municipality can't raise the monthly sewer rate without providing notice and an opportunity to appeal. Stating it as simply as I can, the Obamacare mandate will inevitably force the managed-care insurance industry and the states to defend their use of the Enrollee Hold Harmless clause to deny enrollees a personal and private doctor-patient relationship, as well as their right to access and contract "necessary and appropriate" health care outside the interference of a state-actor insurance company. Furthermore, it's a constitutional review that the states and the insurance industry cannot hope to win.

Already Well-Decided:

While the U. S. Constitution does not set forth an explicit individual right to health care, and the Supreme Court has never interpreted it as providing any such right, this is more a result of the issue having been raised only in the context of an individual's right to receive health care when they cannot afford to pay for it. In other words, the issue has always been raised in terms of government's obligation to provide health care rather than an individual's right to purchase it. Or as the Congressional Research Service stated, "*The question becomes, not whether one has a right to health care that one can pay for, but whether the government or some other entity has an obligation to provide such care to those who cannot afford it.*" (*Health Care Constitutional Rights and Legislative Powers*, Kathleen Swendiman, July 2012). Simply stated, once the context is changed to the right of an individual to access and contract for health care at their own expense, we have an entirely different situation. The right to access health care at one's own expense attaches to a host of Supreme Court decisions and well-established constitutional rights that are simply assumed in the Congressional Research Service's report.

First and foremost in understanding why the right to access health care at one's own expense has never been litigated is the obvious question of who would ever believe that an individual can be denied the right to pay for their own health care? After all, we certainly know that we have a protected right to purchase anything else that is legally available for sale. If a dealer puts a tractor on sale, the law requires the dealer to sell it to whoever offers to buy it. Or, if you or I wish to buy house, we can be confident of our right to purchase it so long as we are willing to pay the advertised price. And, of course, if you order a meal in a restaurant, you can be certain of being served so long as you are willing to pay for the meal. It's not just our system, it's an inseparable part of our American heritage and our well-delineated constitutional rights.

In West Coast Hotel Co. v. Parrish (293 U.S.), the U. S. Supreme Court stated that *"The Constitution does not speak of freedom of contract, it speaks of liberty and prohibits the deprivation of liberty without due process of law."* This simple statement in a landmark case on the right of contract speaks volumes on an enrollee's right to *"due process of law."* That's because enrollees in managed-care health plans are, by state action, deliberately denied their ability to access "necessary and appropriate" health care without: 1.) any notice of this loss of liberty or freedom of contract, 2.) any signed acceptance of the loss, and 3.) any ownership in what is fraudulently promoted as *their* plan. In short, there can be no credible claim of receiving "due process of law" when enrollees are deliberately kept in the dark about their loss and denied any direct participation in a managed-care health plan. And, since the *"essential limitation of liberty in general governs freedom of contract in particular"* (once again West Coast Hotel Co. v. Parrish), I argue that it is well held by the U. S. Supreme Court that no amount of arguing can justify the states' secret and deliberate interference with an enrollee's right to contract health care through their own personal and private doctor-patient relationship in order to promote the interests of a private health insurance market in which enrollees are allowed neither ownership nor informed consent.

In Goldberg v. Kelley (397 U.S.) the Supreme Court ruled that residents of New York City who received financial aid under a federally assisted program of Aid to Families with Dependent Children (AFDC) or under New York State's Home Relief Program could not be dropped from the program without first receiving *"due process of law,"* which must include a *"pre-termination evidentiary hearing*." In doing so the Court stated that "*For qualified recipients, welfare provides the only means to obtain essential food, clothing, housing and medical care. The crucial factor is that the termination of aid might deprive an eligible recipient of the very means by which to live*." In essence, a state's financial concerns cannot supersede a recipient's right to "*due process of law*" when the issue concerns an individual's "*very means by which to live*," which includes "*medical care*."

In Washington v. Harper (494 U.S.) the Supreme Court ruled that "*The Due Process Clause*" of the 14th Amendment "*permits the State to treat a prison inmate who has a serious mental illness with antipsychotic drugs against his will, if he is dangerous to himself or others and the treatment is in his medical interests*." Furthermore, the Court once again made it abundantly clear that an evidentiary hearing must precede such forced treatment wherein the state must prove the treatment is "*medically appropriate*" and the prisoner must be given an "*opportunity to be heard*." In essence, a State's concern for safety within a prison cannot supersede a recipient's right to "*due process of law*" when the issue concerns the determination of their "*medically appropriate*" care.

In Griswold v. Connecticut (544 U.S.) the issue before the Court was whether a state's ban on the use of contraceptives violated the right to marital privacy. In writing for the majority, Justice William O. Douglas wrote that the Bill of Right's specific guarantees have "*penumbras*" created by "*emanations from these guarantees that help give them life and opinion*." In other words, the *spirit* of the First Amendment (free speech), Third Amendment (prohibition on the forced quartering of troops), Fourth Amendment (freedom from searches and seizures), Fifth Amendment (freedom from self-incrimination), and Ninth Amendment (other rights) as applied to the states by the Fourteenth Amendment, creates a general "*right to privacy*" that cannot be unduly infringed. This right to privacy is "*fundamental*" when it affects the relationship of marriage because it "*is of such character that it cannot be denied without violating those fundamental principles of liberty and justice which lie at the base of our civil and political institutions.*" Furthermore, this particular Connecticut law "*seeks to achieve its goals by means of having a maximum destructive impact upon the relationship*" of marriage. Therefore, "**Such a law cannot stand in light of the familiar principle, so often applied by this Court, that a government purpose to control or prevent activities constitutionally subject to state regulation may not be achieved by means which sweep unnecessarily broadly and thereby invade the area of protected freedoms.**"

Then there is Roe v. Wade (410 U.S.). While there is arguably no more disputed Supreme Court ruling, the dispute rests on the issue of abortion. If one simply replaces the word *abortion* with the broader term *health care*, the logic for the dispute vanishes. In essence, while one can logically dispute the Court's reasoning in ruling a woman's right to an abortion is a constitutionally protected right, one cannot logically claim that the reasoning is flawed if applied to all "necessary and appropriate" health care. Even The Heritage Foundation in denouncing the Roe v. Wade decision acknowledged that the Due Process Clause was "*meant to protect the citizens from government abuse by ensuring that no one be deprived of life, liberty, or property except by fair process.*" (Heritage.org/ initiatives/rule-of-law).

Is there anyone who would even attempt to claim that access to "necessary and appropriate" health care at one's own expense involves anything less than "*life*" and "*liberty*"? Or can anyone reasonably dispute that in order to exercise that right of "access" to "necessary and appropriate" health care, one must have an equally protected right to a personal and private contractual relationship with one's own doctor, i.e., a personal and private doctor-patient relationship? "*All these factors the woman and her responsible physician necessarily will consider in consultation.*" (Roe v. Wade).

The point to be taken from all of these cases is that the U. S. Supreme Court has been uniquely consistent in their support of The Heritage Foundation's assertion that the Due Process Clause was "*meant to protect the citizens from government abuse by ensuring that no one be deprived of life, liberty, or property except by fair process."* Using the Court's own words concerning its consistency in past decisions, *"These decisions make it clear that only personal rights that can be deemed "fundamental" or "implicit in the concept of ordered liberty are included in this guarantee of personal privacy." Going back perhaps as far as Union Pacific R. Co. v. Botsford (141 U.S., in 1891) the Court recognized that a right of personal privacy, or a guarantee of certain areas or zones of privacy, does exist under the Constitution."* And, *"This right of privacy, whether it be founded in the Fourteenth Amendment's concept of personal liberty and restrictions upon state action or in the Ninth Amendment's reservation of rights to the people, is broad enough to encompass a woman's decision whether or not to terminate her pregnancy. The determent that the State would impose upon the pregnant woman by denying this choice altogether is apparent."*

The inescapable conclusion is that we need only apply the above decisions of the Court to the right of an enrollee to a private and personal doctor-patient relationship in accessing "necessary and appropriate" health care that an enrollee is willing to pay for, to understand that the U. S. Supreme Court has already ruled on the issue. In essence, we need only exchange the question of a woman's right to an abortion that she is willing to pay for with the right of an individual to the "necessary and appropriate" health care that they are willing to pay for to understand why managed-care health insurance is so blatantly unconstitutional!

And, as if the above cases were not enough to make the case for due process, U. S. District Court Judge Anna J. Brown just ruled on June 24, 2014 that the federal government's practice of putting passengers on a no-fly list violates their constitutional right to due process. Judge Brown concluded: *"Without proper notice and an opportunity to be heard, an individual could be doomed to indefinite placement on the No-Fly List"* and that *"there is nothing"* in the government's administrative procedures *"that remedies this fundamental deficiency"* (The Wall Street Journal, June 25, 2014)

Here we have a ruling that involves national security and even here we have a federal judge ruling that a person's constitutional right to due process cannot be swept aside. The government cannot strip an individual of this fundamental right to *notice and an opportunity to be heard* even for what it views as an issue of national security. How much stronger then is the case of the enrollee who is doomed to be forever without a private and personal doctor-patient relationship that he or she depends on for life itself while being intentionally denied ANY *"notice and . . . opportunity to be heard?"* How much stronger is the case of the enrollee who is doomed to be forever without the freedom to access health care that he or she needs and is willing to pay for? As attorney Shayana Kadidal with the Center for Constitutional Rights in New York has argued, *"Some sort of fair process must exist to challenge such a significant limit on freedom."*

....

SEVEN

> *"Don't interfere with anything in
> the Constitution. That must be
> maintained, for it is the only
> safeguard of our liberties:"*
>
> Abraham Lincoln

Tortious Interference with Contract

Quoting a description of Tortious Interference with Contract from the Harvard Law Review, Vol. 41, No. 6, Apr 1928, Page 728, A *"third person may induce one of the parties to the contract to break his contract"* and to *"interfere by doing some act, which makes performance more burdensome, or impossible, or renders performance of less or no value to the person entitled to it."*

While Tortious Interference with Contract has been and continues to be primarily a state cause of action, it is part of a natural evolution of charges that the Obamacare mandate will force the managed-care insurance industry to address in federal court. Not because it creates some new cause of action, but because it exposes the policies and practices of the insurance industry to federal requirements for disclosure, along with other federal charges, that can be merged with this state cause of action and properly brought in federal court. And once insurers have to disclose the effect their provider contracts and Enrollee Hold Harmless clause have on an enrollee's doctor-patient relationship and access to "necessary and appropriate" health care, a charge of Tortious Interference with Contract becomes both obvious and a prima facie case. After all, the *"inducement to ration care is the very point of any HMO scheme"* and no *"HMO organization could survive without some incentive connecting physician reward with treatment rationing"* and *"the profit incentive to ration care"* goes *"to the very point of any HMO scheme."* (Justice David H. Souter, U. S. Supreme Court Unanimous Decision in Pegram et al. v. Herdrich, 2000). Furthermore, managed-care insurers use a single provider contract to serve <u>all</u> forms of managed-care insurance. Consequently, given the Supreme Court's decision in Pegram and the clarity of the language in the insurer's provider contracts, the only question for a court is whether the act of secretly denying an enrollee's doctor <u>all</u> compensation unless the doctor accepts the insurer's decision on care as well as severing any *"contrary agreement"* an enrollee would reasonably believe they have with *their* doctor or hospital, qualifies as Tortious Interference with Contract. Here again, the individual mandate in Obamacare makes the issue just that simple.

The word *tort* comes from the Latin term *torquere*, which means "twisted or wrong." Its roots date back to Roman law and more recently to English Common Law. It has evolved over the years and exists today in U. S. law as a body of rights, obligations, and remedies to address a broad range of wrongful and damaging civil conduct by serving four objectives. *"First, it seeks to compensate victims for injuries suffered by the culpable actions or inaction of others. Second, it seeks to shift the cost of such injuries to the person or persons who are legally responsible. Third, it seeks to discourage injurious, careless, and risky behavior in the future. Fourth, it seeks to vindicate legal rights and interests that have been compromised, diminished, or emasculated."* See <u>www.legal-dictionary.thefreedictionary.com/Tort+Law.</u>

Tortious Interference with Contract is the part of United States tort law that is specifically designed to address a third party's wrongful interference in a contractual or business relationship. And, because tort law is an area of the law reserved for the states, there are some differences in how the individual states have constructed their laws. However, we are once again blessed by both the clarity of the insurance industry's interference in an enrollee's doctor-patient relationship and the egregious misrepresentation and fraud that they have used to hide their unauthorized interference. In other words, we can leave the details of the differences in state law to the lawyers and focus on the preponderance of evidence that satisfies the letter of the law in most states and the spirit of the law in all cases. This approach is supported by a treatise published by the American Law Institute that summarizes the principles of tort law in the United States. Entitled the "Restatement (Second) of Torts" and adopted by states like Pennsylvania, New York, and Florida, section §766 summarizes the elements of law that are required for a valid charge of Tortious Interference with Contract in the United States. These elements are: *"(1) the existence of a contractual or prospective contractual relation between the complainant and a third party; (2) purposeful action on the defendant, specifically intended to harm the existing relation, or to prevent a prospective relation from occurring; (3) the absence of privilege or justification on the part of the defendant; and (4) the occasioning of actual damage as a result of the defendant's conduct."* See Crivelli v. General Motors Corp., 215 F.3d 386, 344, (2000).

An Existing Contractual Relationship:

The U. S. Supreme Court has carefully and rightfully avoided any decision that could be interpreted as giving an individual a constitutional right to health care. Instead, it and the nation's lower courts have depended on the sanctity and integrity of the doctor-patient relationship and the freedom it provides to access needed health care. In fact, this support for the doctor-patient relationship is so longstanding and obvious that it defies the need to be defended. It is obvious to all that *"a person going to a doctor for treatment impliedly contracts with him for treatment."* (Brown v. Moore, 247

F.2d 711 (3rd Cir. 1957), certiorari denied 78 S. Ct. 148, 355 U. S. 882, 2 L.Ed.2d 112 (Interpreting Pennsylvania law on the contractual relationship between doctor and patient). Furthermore, the relationship created is a *"fiduciary relationship."* (The Law, Science and Public Health site), wherein the *"patient must necessarily place great reliance, faith and confidence in the professional word, advice and acts of the physician."* (Witherell v. Weimer, 421 NE2d 869). Or as the American Medical Association has summarized it, *"Once the relationship has been established, patients should be confident that they are receiving the best medical care physicians can provide, uncompromised by external factors."* ("Report of the Council on Ethical and Judicial Affairs," 1-A-01, AMA, 2001).

Fortunately, the administrative practices of modern medicine make the existence of a doctor-patient relationship easy to prove.

1.) Enrollees are typically required to complete and sign a range of forms and agreements when they establish a doctor-patient relationship. For example, most enrollees are required to: a.) Complete a detailed medical history, b.) Sign some form of power of attorney to allow the doctor to share the enrollee's confidential health information with other health care providers and the enrollee's insurance company, and c.) Sign an agreement accepting responsibility for paying whatever the insurer fails to pay.

2.) It's a rare managed-care plan that does not require its enrollees to pay some amount of "copay" or "coinsurance" for a doctor's services. This means that in language specifically approved by the insurer, the state, and the doctor that the enrollee is a full partner in the purchase of health care. Consequently, on the very face of this approved wording, a typical enrollee must be seen as providing the required consideration for a traditional contract relationship.

3.) The Enrollee Hold Harmless clause specifically states that the doctor must agree that the clause *"supersedes any oral or written contrary agreement now existing or hereafter entered into between Doctor and Subscriber"* (enrollee) and that "*Any attempts to change, amend or waive this provision are void.*" Again relying on the insurer's own words and the wording that the state and the physician have approved, all three parties can be shown to have acknowledged the existence of an "*agreement*" between an in-network doctor and an enrollee — an agreement that can only be a valid doctor-patient relationship as there is no attempt by the parties to describe it as anything else.

Deliberate Interference:

In order to establish deliberate interference, we need to answer two questions. First, does the act of the insurance company interfere with the performance of an enrollee's doctor-patient relationship? And second, is the act intended to damage the enrollee's doctor-patient relationship?

Any time that a third party intercedes in a contractual or business relationship by severing the ability of a contracting party to appropriately compensate a contracted party, there can only be egregious interference with the relationship. In fact, unless the contracting party is free to pay for the services the contracted party is to provide, there can be no valid contract as a matter of law. "*To create an enforceable contract, there must also be a consideration, i.e., each side must receive something of value.*" (¶1005.2, *Lawyer's Desk Book*, 11ᵗʰ Edition). Consequently, the answer to the first question can only be that the insurer's unauthorized interference in an enrollee's doctor-patient relationship effectively severs a relationship that enrollees literally look to for life itself.

As to whether this interference is intentional, we need look only at the insurer's conduct to get our answer. For, if the Enrollee Hold Harmless clause was simply an insolvency provision and/or a provision to prevent balanced billing as insurers would have us believe, they could simply state so in their provider contracts. They could include wording something like, "*This provision is limited to instances of insurer insolvency and/or balanced billing by a provider.*" But they don't. Instead they allow the all-too-clear language of the

Enrollee Hold Harmless clause to stand without limits, hidden within confidential provider contracts and misrepresented in the few instances where the language is called into question. Consequently, the answer to the second question on deliberate interference can only be that the army of knowledgeable attorneys employed by the managed-care insurance industry knows exactly what their use of the Enrollee Hold Harmless clause does to an enrollee's doctor-patient relationship as well as the role it plays in the industry's rationing of health care outside the view of enrollees and the public.

No Authority to Act and Hide:

The answer here is a pure joy for this non-attorney. Even I know that one cannot be held accountable for an agreement they have never seen, let alone signed. And this is where I get to extract some comic relief from the mess the managed-care insurance industry has created — their veritable house of cards.

To eliminate their vulnerability to a charge of Tortious Interference of Contract, insurers *could* simply have their enrollees sign a policy or an agreement accepting the insurer's use of the Enrollee Hold Harmless clause. In fact, this very suggestion was made by the U. S. Justice Department during the Clinton administration and again as a proposal of the National Academy for State Health Policy as part of their State Coverage Initiatives. However, to make such a change, insurers would have to disclose the terms and conditions under which they ration health care as well as their use of the Enrollee Hold Harmless clause. But such disclosure would open insurers to a range of charges and litigation that boggles the mind. On the other hand, if they elect to have enrollees sign such an agreement and not disclose the terms and conditions under which they ration care or how they apply the Enrollee Hold Harmless clause, the signatures are unenforceable, and they open themselves to a charge of criminal fraud. It's literally the house of cards they deserve. Or, more appropriately stated, insurers lack any and all authority to interfere in an enrollee's doctor-patient relationship because enrollees have been given *zero* ownership in their managed-care plan. Consequently, insurers have found themselves with no choice but to carefully and deliberately hide their interference in our private and personal doctor-patient relationship.

The All Too Real Damage to Enrollees:

The damage done to enrollees is far more extensive than one might initially think. This is because the damage stems from more than twenty years of interference and at least three separate areas of loss:

Loss of the Doctor-Patient Relationship Itself:

There is probably no relationship in society that an enrollee values more than the one he or she has with their personal physician or the physician to whom they have entrusted the health of their children. It's a value and matter of an enrollee's property that society promotes, the courts have long supported, and the future must ensure. For without this vital right of ownership, there can be no freedom to access necessary health care. Just as the loss of the right to an attorney would mean the loss of one's freedom to access justice through the courts.

Forced to Accept a Lower Standard of Care:

Any reasonable research into the policies and practices of modern-day managed-care health insurance will reveal the subtle, but clear, substitution of the lowest cost average standard of care as determined by an insurer for the best available care as determined by an attending physician. In one way or other, it's a loss we have all experienced. Your doctor prescribes an MRI but your insurer insists on a less expensive x-ray. Or your doctor is prescribing surgery and your insurer is insisting on less costly medication. These are losses that are not only all too common, but largely unseen and only possible through the interference in our doctor-patient relationship.

Loss from Fraudulent Billings:

As I have pointed out repeatedly, the billing requirements

for managed-care health insurance force in-network doctors to bill an enrollee only *after* billing the insurer. The insurer then examines the bill, denies some charges, bundles some individual charges to reduce the amount of the bill, accepts some charges, applies the discounted prices from the insurer's provider contract, applies the deduction from any applicable co-insurance, deductible, or cap, and then issues a payment significantly less than the physician's bill. The physician must then appeal this underpayment or surrender the right to appeal. The doctor then bills the enrollee for whatever the doctor claims is a correct and enforceable bill. The insurer and the only party in possession of the information needed to define an enforceable bill simply walks away from the issue, i.e., leaves the enrollee to the mercy of a doctor's billing office and collection process. Furthermore, this is a billing office that: 1.) Believes it is being routinely and unfairly denied appropriate payment by the insurer, 2.) Lacks the information needed to make a billing legally enforceable, 3.) Is barred from disclosing such billing information even if they happen to have it available, and 4.) Knows that the insurer *must* refuse to help an enrollee determine a correct and enforceable bill or risk disclosing its use of the Enrollee Hold Harmless clause and their infringement of the doctor-patient relationship.

The bottom line is that the billing scheme created by managed-care health insurance is so complex that it defies the requirements for a legally enforceable bill. In addition, the complexity of the system places enrollees at the mercy of commercial billing agents. Billing agents who have every reason to inflate a doctor's bill beyond what neither the doctor's provider contract nor the law allows. And, while the actual wording of the Enrollee Hold Harmless clause may vary a bit from state to state, these small differences can be very significant when it comes to determining a legally enforceable bill. Because the Enrollee Hold Harmless clause is worded to provide an absolute bar against billing an enrollee, the only charges that can be legally billed to an enrollee are the specific items permitted by the Enrollee Hold Harmless clause contained in a doctor's provider contract. Or stating the issue more simply, the wording of the Enrollee Hold Harmless clause places very clear limits on what a doctor can and cannot bill to an enrollee. So, as my friend the judge said, *"When you use one contract for multiple uses"* (the many different managed-care plans), *"you have something that doesn't address any of its uses."* And so it is with the insurance industry's provider contracts. One set of limits on what a doctor can bill, but countless plans with widely different coverage.

My point here is not to vilify physicians but to show the difference between what an in-network physician believes is fair compensation for his or her services and what his or her provider contract and the law allow them to bill an enrollee. In most cases these are very different values. And they have been so for more than twenty years. In fact, in fairness to the insurance companies, the issue has become so convoluted and complex that I doubt that even the largest insurers know how to calculate a legally enforceable bill that is free of controversy. But then again, they are solely responsible for creating the mess. Even worse, insurers have used the issue to line their pockets at the expense of both physicians and the public.

Punitive Damages and Injunctive Relief:

I am more than willing to leave these considerations to sharp minds in the legal community. However, I will point out that the serious nature of both the deliberate infringement of the doctor-patient relationship and the fraudulent bills that flow from this infringement justify not only punitive damages, but injunctive relief as well. In fact, the justification for injunctive relief is another factor in why Heritage, conservatives and the Republican Party are so opposed to Obamacare. I just wish they were as committed to disclosure and protecting the rights of the individual as they are to repealing Obamacare. See my letters to U. S. Senators Burr, Coburn and Hatch at the back of the book (Appendix 12).

EIGHT

....

"The least initial deviation from the ruth is multiplied later a thousand old:"

Aristotle

The Mother of All Class Actions

When the states adopted the National Association of Insurance Commissioners' (NAIC's) HMO Model Act in the 1990s, they could not have anticipated the countless plans and options the insurance industry would create in pursuit of lower costs and higher profits in an increasingly complex market. Consequently, it's only fair to assume that they had little or no idea of the limits they were placing on their future plans or how their actions would forever change the landscape of our nation's health care delivery system.

In the 1990s the states were primarily focused on preserving their right to regulate health insurance, particularly in cases of HMO insolvency. As a result, they paid little attention to the limits they were placing on what a provider could legally bill to an enrollee ten or twenty years in the future. Furthermore, since the states' primary goal was to deny providers the right to sue enrollees in instances of insurer insolvency, they were focused on defining what a provider could not bill to an enrollee rather than what a provider could legally bill to an enrollee. It would also be fair to say that the lobbyists for the insurance industry had the same focus. Add in the fact that the states felt compelled to adopt much of the National Association of Insurance Commissioners' lengthy HMO Model Act, and we can begin to understand how the states established such extensive requirements for provider contracts. All viewed as simple and reasonable requirements when they were adopted. However, time never stands still, and it certainly hasn't here.

Because insurers were required to establish a detailed state-approved contract with each of their in-network providers, large insurers were faced with an enormous task as well as a very expensive one. These insurers had literally tens of thousands of individual contracts to complete. So in keeping with their practice of streamlining operations to cut costs, insurers chose to established one contract for each provider and to renew it no more often than necessary. Whether these were conscious decisions or merely the result of inaction we will never know. But what we can say is that the insurance industry exists today with one approved contract per provider for all their constantly changing plans, products, and options — a contract with an Enrollee Hold Harmless clause that was written twenty or so years ago. As a result, the industry (insurers, providers, and the states) is saddled with provider contracts that no longer fit the complex billing requirements of today's insurance market. In fact, I am quite confident that if a sharp attorney were to compare what provider contracts and state laws allow a hospital to bill an enrollee, with what hospitals have actually billed enrollees, they would discover a pattern of overcharging, misrepresentation, and fraud dating back some ten or even twenty years. Or, more simply, the attorney would discover the "mother" of all class action lawsuits.

Consider the example of Pennsylvania. As best as I can determine, neither the provider contracts approved by the state nor the laws and regulations of the Commonwealth of Pennsylvania allow a provider to bill an enrollee for a deductible or a cap or even coinsurance for an item an insurer has denied for coverage. And that is just the start of the problems the health care industry has created for itself.

In Texas, Title 28, Part 1, Chapter 11, Subchapter J, Rule §11.901 states that the only exceptions to the Enrollee Hold Harmless Clause are for the collection of *"supplemental charges or copayments made in accordance with the terms of (applicable agreement) between HMO and enrollee."* And, since *"supplemental charges"* refer to charges for additional services which are "non-covered services" that fall outside an applicable provider agreement, the law in Texas and their provider agreements appear to absolutely bar providers from billing enrollees for anything other than an appropriate *"copayment."* Furthermore, the term *applicable agreement* assumes that there is some form of an agreement *"between HMO and enrollee"* when there is no such agreement. Managed-care operates without any signed agreement between an enrollee and his or her insurer. So there is *no* "applicable agreement."

These are but two examples of how the states have failed to keep up with the needs of an ever changing market. However, even where states have done a better job, there is a significant gap between what a provider can legally bill and what they have been billing enrollees for years.

Because applicable state laws and the Enrollee Hold Harmless clause were written ten to twenty years ago, there has been little or no attempt to ensure that their limitations on billing match the requirements of the current managed-care insurance system. Furthermore, given the success of the industry's long-standing policy of allowing enrollees to believe that they own their plan and that anything their insurer fails to pay is the enrollee's responsibility, there really hasn't been a problem for the industry.

The difference between what providers needed to bill and what they were legally allowed to bill developed slowly. In addition, the aggressive billing practices of modern mega-hospitals is only a recent phenomenon. Hospitals have gotten *"more aggressive because they now know that so much more of the bill is going to go uncovered.*" (Sara Rosenbaum, George Washington University Law School and former advisor to President Bill Clinton, Huffington Post, May 2012). And, "*When a hospital doesn't get paid as much as it wants from one source, it tries to make up the difference in other ways.*" (Robert Huckman, Harvard Business School, Huffington Post, May 2013).

By the time the insurance industry became aware of the problem, the die had already been cast. To correct their provider contracts, the industry would have to ask states to change both their laws and the Enrollee Hold Harmless clause. However, to do that, they would have to explain why the change was necessary. And to do that, they would risk disclosing years of overbilling enrollees as well as the use of the Enrollee Hold Harmless clause to ration health care. Both of these are disclosures the insurance industry simply cannot afford. Furthermore, such changes would involve discussions that the states can't afford to touch with a ten foot pole.

The solution to the problem has actually proven to be quite simple. Insurers have simply gotten out of the way and allowed their in-network hospitals and other in-network providers to bill enrollees as they see fit. To quote an attorney for Blue Cross in my litigation against the Enrollee Hold Harmless clause, "*We would simply let them pay.*" And that is exactly what the managed-care insurance industry has done. Rather than fulfill their ERISA duty to explain what a provider can and cannot bill an enrollee and take responsibility for a billing that is theirs as a matter of law, insurers have put as much distance as they can between themselves and what their providers actually bill enrollees. Unfortunately for enrollees, it's a solution that works for both insurers and their in-network providers, particularly hospitals.

I'm stressing hospitals because that is where the big money is. Where a bill from a doctor might add up to hundreds of dollars, hospital bills can easily run into the hundreds of thousands of dollars. These are the bills that drive families from their homes and into bankruptcy. It's the old axiom of "*follow the money.*" Your doctor's bill may be an inconvenience, but an unexpected hospital bill can cost you everything you own. In essence, hospital bills are where enrollees have been fleeced for years. It's also an area where the insurance industry and the states, have deliberately turned a blind eye.

The Dependence on Naïve and Trusting Enrollees:

To properly understand this issue of deliberate overbilling, we need to begin by understanding that regardless of what insurers and their in-network doctors, hospitals, other providers of health care services, collection services, and employers would have us believe, the bills from an in-network provider are *not* an enrollee's responsibility. As a matter of both contract and law, they are the responsibility of an enrollee's primary managed-care insurance company. This is an extremely important point, because it's exactly the opposite of how the system has been allowed to operate and what *enrollees have been encouraged to believe*.

Following an enrollee's discharge, the hospital bills the enrollee's insurer as it must under the laws of every state. The insurer then reviews the bill, declines charges they believe are improperly billed, declines all charges they alone find to be for care that is not "necessary and appropriate," bundles charges where they believe the hospital has inflated the cost of care, and then applies the negotiated rates contained in the hospital's provider contract to the charges that remain. Then they deduct and coinsurance, copayments or deductibles. Then, and only then, they forward their approved and adjusted payment to the hospital. The hospital then sends the enrollee a bill that is essentially limited to: 1.) The hospital's unadjusted bill, 2.) A figure the hospital claims is what the insurer should pay, 3.) The amount the insurer has paid, and 4.) The difference between these last two amounts being what the hospital claims is the "responsibility" of the enrollee. It's all so simple. In fact, the hospital will almost certainly claim they have left out the bothersome details that went into calculating their bill because enrollees *don't want to receive all that confusing and frustrating information*.

The best analogy that I can think of is grocery shopping for a large Thanksgiving dinner. You arrive at the checkout counter with an overflowing cart. After the clerk scans all the items in the cart, you get a bill that only lists an undiscounted total and a discounted total that they claim you owe. There is no list of items or individual prices. Absolutely no indication of whether you got the sale price for the twenty-pound turkey or whether what's in the cart matches what you are being billed. And, of course, you are assured by the clerk that the missing information is being withheld solely for your convenience.

Understanding the Problem:

I have chosen to repeat the grocery analogy because it is actually very close to what enrollees experience following a lengthy stay in a hospital. Like the bill for a large amount of groceries, a hospital bill is comprised of a long list of individual charges for the services and products that have been supplied over the enrollee's hospitalization. The charges come from a price list that is typically referred to as a Chargemaster. This is a published list that contains the hospital's pricing for thousands of individually coded services and products. However, these are not the prices an enrollee needs to receive to understand their bill. The prices an enrollee needs are the ones the insurer has negotiated with the hospital for use with the enrollee's plan, i.e., the prices contained in the hospital's provider contract, *which the insurer will not disclose*.

But the problem gets worse. Because insurers are free to deny any of a hospital's long list of individual charges and bundle those it believes reduces the cost of care, an enrollee needs to receive the details of each and every decision their insurer makes on each and every individual charge to understand a hospital bill. This is because, whenever an insurer denies coverage for a particular item, the hospital can't bill the charge for that item to an enrollee. And if the hospital can't bill it, there can't be any co-insurance and it can't be included in any calculation of a deductible or cap. Furthermore, an appeal of any such denial or bundling is solely the responsibility of the hospital, regardless of how vigorously anyone states otherwise. In fact, the hospital is the only one with the information and knowledge needed to appeal an insurer's denial of payment or bundling of charges. This is particularly true when an insurer denies coverage because the hospital has failed to properly document a charge for an item or service.

The Hospital's Problem:
To be fair to in-network hospitals, the billing scheme that managed-care insurers have created is so complex that I would readily agree that it's next to impossible for a hospital to create an accurate bill. Consequently, it should not be surprising that hospitals have adjusted their billing procedures to solve the problem. They simply ignore individual denials of coverage by a primary insurer and bill enrollees for the difference between what the hospital believes an insurer should have paid and what the insurer actually paid. The hospital then ignores any secondary insurance and bills the enrollee, claiming that the unpaid difference is the enrollee's "responsibility." This is a misrepresentation and intentional fraud created by the best minds in the legal profession.

By claiming that the unpaid balance is the responsibility of the enrollee, the hospital: 1.) Preserves an argument that it hasn't actually billed an enrollee in violation of state law and its provider contract, 2.) Creates the possibility that the enrollee will simply pay the unpaid balance, and 3.) Establishes an enrollee's responsibility for the unpaid balance that can be readily pursued in a collection process and the courts. The best part is that the trusting and unsophisticated enrollee can be counted on to respond slowly, if at all, making a hospital's inflated bill more enforceable with each passing day. In order to take advantage of the protections available under the federal Fair Debt Collection Practices Act (15 U.S.C. 1601 et seq) an enrollee must formally dispute the validity of a bill within thirty days of the receipt of a bill, or else the collection agency may assume that the debt is valid and subject to collection [15 USC

1692g(3)].

An Enrollee's Right to Understand a Bill:

Rather than cite chapter and verse of an enrollee's right to understand a bill generated by an in-network hospital, we need only read the printed handout that patients get when they enter a hospital. This little handout lists all a patient's rights and responsibilities. Every one of these printed handouts that I have ever seen states in very clear terms that a patient has a right to understand his or her bill. In fact, the law allows nothing less. Consequently, the issue isn't whether enrollees have a right to understand their hospital bill. It's knowing what to request.

The following is my suggestion for an enrollee's response to a hospital bill believed to be in excess of what should be owed. I believe it's self-explanatory.

From: Managed-care Enrollee
To: Hospital Billing Office

Subject: My right to understand the bill I just received

I have received your bill and need to remind you that the law and the provider contract that you have signed with my insurance company severely limit what you can bill me, regardless of any failure of my insurance company to pay for my care. Furthermore, because: 1.) Your bill is computed from a long list of individually coded and priced items taken from what I believe you refer to as your Chargemaster, 2.) I have a right to know the prices for each of these items that are listed in the provider contract that you have signed with my insurance company, 3.) My insurance company has the authority to deny or bundle any and all of your individual charges in order to reduce the overall amount of your bill, 4.) Any individual charge or group of charges that my insurance company elects to deny, for whatever reason, cannot be billed to me nor can it be used in computing any co-insurance, deductible, or cap, 5.) The application of any co-insurance, deductible, or cap requires a detailed explanation of items 1 through 4 as well as information you can obtain only from my insurance company, and 6.) Any appeal of my insurance company's denial of charges, bundling and/or failures to pay for whatever reason is solely your responsibility. Consequently, I am requesting the following information as the minimum needed to understand my bill.

1. A complete list of the individual items, codes, and prices from your Chargemaster that comprise your bill.
2. The discounted prices listed in your provider contract for each of these same items.
3. My insurance company's decisions on whether to pay for each of these same items, including any bundling of charges.
4. A detailed accounting of how my insurance company's decisions on payment affect any applicable co-insurance, deductible, and/or cap.
5. A copy of the Enrollee Hold Harmless clause in your provider contract, which defines what you can and cannot bill me.
6. A copy of all other provisions and language in your provider contract that limit what you can bill me.
7. The same above information (1 through 6) for my secondary insurance, when and where applicable.

Because the information I am requesting is no more than: 1.) what is needed to understand my bill, 2.) what your publication on patients' rights and responsibilities promises, and 3.) what the law entitles me to receive, I have to assume that all this information is readily available. If I am wrong or you have a different understanding of any of above, please get back to me, because like you, I want to get you paid and settle this matter as soon as possible.

Sincerely,

One Confused Enrollee

"A brilliant letter! It could be a huge help to people"

A quote from the editor of the book

If I haven't convinced you that there is massive misrepresentation and overbilling of enrollees that dates back at least ten or twenty years, then I am going to be very surprised. Because, while what I have requested in my letter will produce a mind-numbing array of detail that defies interpretation, it's what is needed to compute an accurate hospital bill. Furthermore, it includes facts that cannot be disputed within the system that the states and the managed-care insurance industry have created in law and contract. Furthermore, these are facts that neither the insurance industry nor the states can afford to discuss in public.

A recent experience of my daughter, Kris, can serve to show just how brazen and fraudulent the managed-care billing process can be as well as how fearful insurers are of allowing enrollees to understand what is going on. It's also the only time I have ever seen an insurance company completely out of words and hung twisting on their own petard.

My grandson had spent a short time in a local hospital at a cost $950. To my daughter Kris's surprise, her insurer sent her a check for the $950, along with instructions to use the money to pay the hospital. However, when Kris tried to pay the hospital, they refused the payment. Kris then tried to return the money to the insurance company, but was told that they could not accept her check either. Then, some weeks later, Kris received a notice (not a bill, mind you, but simply a "Notice") from the insurance company claiming she owed them $950. Kris then called the insurer and spoke to a supervisor, who explained that since they could not bill Kris for the $950, they would simply add charges to her future payments until they had recovered the $950. However, when Kris asked whether she would be aware of these additional charges, the supervisor said, *"Probably not. You most likely won't ever see them."*

Fortunately, Kris has full coverage through her employer, so she knew the insurer couldn't simply inflate her future payments. Her plan doesn't require any co-insurance, deductible, or cap. So in Kris's case, the supervisor's threats were hollow. However, the supervisor did all she could to intimidate Kris into sending a $950 check without receiving a bill or any form of written explanation from the insurer.

In a written response, Kris offered to pay the requested amount so long as she received a bill or other written explanation of the debt. The insurer's response has been to simply abandon the $950. They simply refuse to put anything in writing to justify the debt. And failing to do that, they can't enforce the $950 billing. Or to state it more directly, it was safer to write off the $950 than to risk having to explain why the hospital had been unable to accept Kris' check.

Like so many times in my life, God stepped in and gave me a helping hand. Here I was in the middle of writing this book and Kris' insurer provides the perfect example how in-network providers are barred from accepting a direct payment from an enrollee. In Kris' case, the insurer obviously screwed up by sending her the $950 dollars to pay for her son's care rather than sending the payment to the hospital as is required by both Pennsylvania law and the hospital's provider contract. Kris cashed the insurer's check and then sent a personal check for $950 to the hospital. And since the check was now in the form of a personal check from an enrollee, the hospital could only return it. However, since Kris had provided payment and it had been refused, the debt was completely settled.

And here is where we get to the insurer's petard. Because the hospital was barred from accepting Kris' payment and the insurer can't afford to risk disclosing the reach of the Enrollee Hold Harmless clause, neither the hospital nor the insurer can bill Kris for the $950 without accepting significant liability. Furthermore, Kris has rendered payment, so the debt is completely settled. And yes, I'm smiling and Kris has $950 of found money!!!

Rest assured that if either the hospital or the insurer had provided a written explanation of the issue or an appropriate bill, Kris would have paid them in full. In fact, to the best of my knowledge, the $950 is sitting off to the side just in case her insurer or the hospital change their mind and send an appropriate bill.

The points that can be taken from this bizarre example are numerous, but the one intended here is the brazenness of the insurance company supervisor in telling Kris that they would add $950 to her future billings that she would not see. It's a brazenness that can only come from an insurer's ability to routinely inflate bills outside the view or understanding of trusting and naïve enrollees.

Why didn't the insurer just allow Kris to return the $950 when she initially offered to do so? I have to guess that it was because they would have had to account for the payment. By sending Kris the $950 and telling her to pay the hospital, the insurer broke Pennsylvania state law and breached its provider contract with the hospital. In addition, if the insurer allowed Kris to document the return of the $950, they would be documenting the inability of the hospital to accept Kris's payment for her son's health care — something I failed to get this very insurance company to acknowledge in ten years of litigation.

Another example of fraudulent billing was described to me just last night at dinner. My wife and I had dinner with two other couples, and one of the wives happened to be a nurse. She described a recent situation where her father was seriously ill and she had spent a great deal of time monitoring his care and treatment. She further explained that she had demanded a copy of the exact charges that went onto his bill and reviewed each one carefully. She found $15,000 worth of charges for things he never received — charges deliberately included to fraudulently inflate what the hospital could bill her father.

For those who might argue that this could be the result of simple billing errors rather that a system of deliberate fraud, please keep in mind that an entire business has developed around analyzing hospital bills for the very things my dinner companion found on her father's bill. For the better part of $100 an hour, organizations like Medical Bills Auditing Service (MBAA) will take a hospital bill and do exactly what my friend the nurse did for her father. They demand a full accounting of the charges billed and then review each one for appropriateness, given a patient's specific course of treatment and reasonable hospital expenses. The success of these businesses demonstrates that the inflation of hospital bills is systemic and not a random scattering of billing errors.

Equally Free to Exploit the System:

This brings me to one of the most unrecognized but ingenious parts of the managed-care system. While insurance companies contractually assign themselves the power to determine an accurate and appropriate bill from a hospital, they keep their determinations to themselves and allow hospitals to essentially bill enrollees as they see fit. In short, insurers use their expertise and contractual authority to determine accurate hospital charges but then ignore their fiduciary duty to share this information with their enrollees. In fact, they knowingly leave enrollees at the mercy of hospital billing offices and collection agencies.

The underlying issue is that enrollees lack the knowledge needed to audit a hospital bill. Furthermore, they certainly can't be expected to know everything they did or did not receive while in a hospital — things that in the case of my friend the nurse totaled $15,000 worth of items and services her father never received. The point is that enrollees receive a hospital bill that only their insurer and doctor are capable of auditing and the hospital doesn't even certify as accurate. Furthermore, the insurer gets as far away from the bill as possible, and the doctor has neither the time nor any incentive to audit a bill. And, of course, if an enrollee should happen to find a charge for something that was never received, the hospital has a ready and solid defense. It's simply a regrettable and unintended error made by the hospital's immensely complicated billing system. Or more simply stated from a hospital's perspective, *"Heads we almost always win, and tails we never lose."*

The ingenious part of these fraudulent hospital bills is that in order to hide the use of the Enrollee Hold Harmless clause, insurers need to get as far away from auditing hospital bills for their enrollees as possible. This allows hospitals to inflate their bills essentially as much as they deem appropriate. The result is that both the insurer and the hospital are free to pursue a stronger bottom line while the enrollee picks up the tab. Even better, if, by some outside chance, an overbilling is found, there is no one or organization that can be held accountable.

An Excellent Example in Case Law:

While court rulings that support strict limits on what a hospital can legally bill to an enrollee are few and far between, there is a case that was heard by the Wisconsin Court of Appeals in 1999 that is of particular interest. It's cited as Thomas and Beverly Dorr v. Sacred Heart Hospital, No. 98-1772, in which the court ruled that the *"enrollee hold harmless provision of the Provider Agreement between the hospital and Group Health* (the Dorrs's HMO) *operates to exclude a debt owed the hospital by the Dorrs."* In addition, the court affirmed the applicability of charges against the hospital for false representation, unfair debt collection practices, breach of contract, racketeering, tortious interference with contract, and punitive damages.

The case arose as a result of Sacred Heart Hospital's filing a lien pursuant to Wisconsin state law on proceeds from a liability insurance settlement due Beverly Dorr from an automobile accident. Her health insurer, Group Health Cooperative (an HMO), had a provider contract with Sacred Heart to provide medical services to Group Health's enrollees at an agreed-to discounted rate. Nevertheless, Sacred Heart chose to pursue the undiscounted cost of Beverly's care by filing a lien on the insurance proceeds due the Dorrs from a separate settlement.

Immediately following her automobile accident, Beverly Dorr was taken to Sacred Heart Hospital, where she was admitted and treated for her injuries. Upon her admission, the hospital obtained the Dorrs's insurance information, which indicated that she had full coverage with Group Health. Shortly after her discharge from Sacred Heart, Beverly developed complications and was readmitted to the hospital. As with her first hospitalization, she was fully covered by her insurance with Group Health. The total cost of the two hospitalizations was $27,051.65. However, in accordance with the rates Sacred Heart had agreed to in its provider contract, Sacred Heart could only bill Group Health $17,618.

The driver of the other car in the accident was insured by Wisconsin American Mutual Insurance Company (WAMIC) for automobile liability, with a $50,000 per person limit. The Dorrs eventually settled their personal injury claim against this other driver and WAMIC for the liability limit of $50,000. Sacred Heart then filed a lien against the Dorrs's settlement for $27,051.65, the original undiscounted bill for Beverly's hospitalization.

I won't bother the reader with the details of the arguments in the case or the detailed analysis done by the court. The essence of it all is that after two separate court reviews, the contractual *"enrollee hold harmless provision of the Provider Agreement between the hospital and Group Health"* was held to *"unambiguously negate the existence of the Dorrs's obligation to pay Sacred Heart."* Or stating it more clearly, the contractual Enrollee Hold Harmless clause in Sacred Heart's provider contract provided an absolute bar against Sacred Heart's billing the Dorrs. Furthermore, the court concluded that there was ample evidence that Sacred Heart acted *"with intentional disregard for the Dorrs's rights."*

The bottom line here is that, as stated by the Wisconsin Appeals Court, *"The clear and unambiguous terms of the Enrollee Hold Harmless Clause create a contractual obligation to hold subscribers harmless for payment for hospital services. The provision's terms are designed specifically for the purpose of protecting HMO subscribers. As such, the HMO subscribers are third-party beneficiaries of this contractual provision, a breach of which supports a third-party beneficiary breach of contract claim."* The court further concluded that when it can be shown that there is a pattern of hospital disregard for enrollees' right to be held harmless, as the court found in the Dorrs's case, the hospital can be pursued for a variety of fraudulent billing practices including RICO and consumer protection laws and subjected to punitive damages.

The importance of the Dorr case is that it provides a detailed analysis of a hospital's contractual obligation under the Enrollee Hold Harmless clause as well as a detailed analysis of the causes of action available to enrollees when hospitals engage in a pattern of disregard for the obligation they owe enrollees under the *"unambiguous terms"* of the Enrollee Hold Harmless clause.

While there are other cases that support a hospital's *"obligation to hold subscribers harmless,"* these other cases largely involve only the enrollee hold-harmless language as it appears in state law. Cases like Samsel v. Allstate in the Supreme Court of Arizona (2002), Gianetti v. Siglinger in the Connecticut Appellate Court (2006), Scull v. Grover in the Court of Appeals of Maryland (2012), and West v. Shelby in the Court of Appeals of Tennessee (2012) all hold that, as a matter of state law, hospitals are barred from billing the enrollees in a managed-care plan for anything other than the few exceptions listed in the law.

And, while the uniformity of these other decisions is important, I believe they pale by comparison to the findings in Dorr v. Sacred Heart. For while the meaning of the language in a particular state statute can be actively debated, as we can see in the case of the Insurance Federation of Pennsylvania v. Commonwealth Insurance Department in the Commonwealth Court of Pennsylvania, the interpretation of contract language presents no such problem. The interpretation of a contract reaches no further than the contract itself. For, if the parties to a provider contract meant to limit or restrict what the Dorr court found to be the clear and unambiguous language of the Enrollee Hold Harmless clause, the parties would surely have included equally clear and unambiguous language limiting the application of the Clause.

A point worth mentioning concerning these other cases is the absence of any reference to the contractual obligation created by the insurers' provider contracts with their mandated Enrollee Hold Harmless clause. However, given that even the U. S. Supreme Court was unaware of these contract obligations when it issued its unanimous ruling in Aetna v. Davila, 542 U.S., I guess it's not too surprising that these lower courts and their attorneys were equally unaware of the limitations imposed by the insurance industry's provider contracts and Enrollee Hold Harmless clause. This is something I can attest to from my own experience with litigating our inability to pay for Sandy's care and the ridicule I received from every attorney I spoke to in the Philadelphia area for even suggesting that we could get a copy of the provider contracts involved the case. I can still hear the attorney from Litvin Blumberg, Philadelphia's largest law firm in health care law, telling me that "*I was crazy if I thought Sandy's insurer would ever surrender copies of its provider contracts. They will never give them up.*" This was one of the reasons the attorney gave for dropping our case as too difficult and costly to pursue. While I was eventually able to prove him wrong in getting access to these provider contracts, it took me more than three years to force the insurer to produce them. And even then, they came as sealed documents that I can never disclose outside of court.

All this speaks directly to the secrecy the insurance industry has created around its provider contracts and their bar on enrollee payments — contracts so secret that even the U. S. Supreme Court wasn't aware of them when it ruled in the landmark case, Aetna v. Devila. Here the Court unanimously ruled that upon the denial of coverage, the enrollee "*could have simply paid for the treatment themselves and then sought reimbursement through a §5029(a)(1) (B) action*" and that the denial of coverage "*under ERISA-regulated benefit plans, fall within the scope of, and are completely pre-empted by, ERISA §5029(a)(1)(B).*" Or to put this unanimous ruling in simple English, the only recourse an enrollee has when denied coverage under a managed-care plan is to pay for the care and then sue the insurer under ERIAS to recover the cost of the care. In other words, the insurance industry's provider contracts and Enrollee Hold Harmless clause are such a well-kept secret that even the U. S. Supreme Court was unaware that its unanimous ruling in Aetna v. Davila was absolutely impossible for an enrollee to accomplish.

In order to "*have simply paid for the treatment themselves,*" the enrollee must *have* the freedom to contract and pay outside the interference of his or her insurer. And, to then sue the insurer for *"reimbursement through a §5029(a)(1)(B) action,"* the enrollee must have actually paid for the care he or she received. However, neither of these are possible under the insurance industry's provider contracts and Enrollee Hold Harmless clause.

And for those who would argue that the Court simply could not be that unaware of these provider contracts and their Enrollee Hold Harmless clause, there are only two possible explanations for its ruling in Aetna v. Devila . First, that the entire Court was willing to provide a ruling that had no relevance to the facts that exist in the nation's managed-care insurance system. Or that the Court, like the rest of us, naturally believed that there is no way under U. S. law that enrollees could be denied the right to pay for their own health care — a fact that took the death of Sandy and ten years of painstaking litigation for me to drag out of the insurance industry.

How Hospitals Falsely Promote "It's Your Bill":

"The Hospital (name omitted) *files insurance claims on patient's behalf. This does not release patients from responsibilities for charges billed to their account. Insurance contracts are between patients and insurance companies. Regardless of the type of insurance, bills are ultimately the responsibility of patients. Any portion of the bill not paid promptly by insurance companies is charged directly to patients ----."*

and

"It is understood that you assume the financial responsibility of paying for all services rendered either through third-party payers (your insurance company) or being personally responsible for payment for any services which are not covered by your insurance policies."

Both of these statements have been copied directly from a printed bulletin given to patients when they are admitted to one of the largest and most prestigious hospitals in the country. And while these are admittedly one of the worst examples of this type misrepresentation that I have come across, they are anything but isolated examples of how enrollees are led to view their hospital bills as solely their responsibility. *"It is understood that you assume the financial responsibility of paying for all services rendered"* — *"You are expected to pay your bills in a timely manner"* — *"You are responsible for assuring that the financial obligations of your health care are fulfilled as promptly as possible"* — You are *"to pay bills promptly to assure that your financial obligations for your health care are fulfilled. Late payments increase overall charges"* — *"You are responsible for the financial costs relating to your care. These costs must be paid in a timely manner"* — *"You are responsible for paying for the hospital care services"* — You are *"To compensate* (the Hospital) *for services provided, including compliance with insurance requirements"* and on and on. In fact I was unable to find a single example of where a hospital made any attempt what-so-ever to acknowledge that their provider contracts contain an absolute bar against billing an enrollee for a *"Covered Service,"* even when the insurer refuses to cover the cost and the enrollee is willing and able to pay for it.

The bottom line is that all of us, including the members of the U. S. Supreme Court, view a hospital bill as our very own financial responsibility, not just because we really can't view it as anything else, but because the hospitals and other providers of managed-care services have taken full advantage of their ability to reinforce this belief and to profit directly from it.

The Inescapable Conclusion:

The inescapable conclusion is that the managed-care insurance industry and their in-network hospitals have hidden the terms contained their provider contracts, inflated their bills and misrepresented the responsibility of enrollees to pay these bills for years. And, they have done so at the direct expense of enrollees.

Whether they have done it purely to enhance profits or to simply streamline their accounting and billing procedures is of no consequence. The only relevant fact is that they have done it knowingly and shown themselves, time and again, willing to mislead even the courts in order to retain their power over unsuspecting enrollees.

One final point. In doing my research for the book, I spoke to numerous people from the health care community. They included doctors, nurses, lawyers, accountants and even a former administrative head of billing for the largest hospital in our area. Not one of them contested my contention that hospital bills sent to enrollees have been, and continue to be, deliberately inflated beyond what is a legally enforceable bill. Not one of them so much as questioned that this misrepresentation and overbilling provides a basis for "The Mother of All Class Actions."

NINE

···......................

*"Organized crime constitutes
nothing more than a guerrilla war
against society:"*

Lyndon B. Johnson

A Rico Action in Waiting

Understanding Rico:

Given the popularity of gangster movies in the United States, most of us are well aware of the efforts of the federal government to rein in organized crime. A key element in those efforts was passage of the Organized Crime Control Act in 1970. Best known simply as RICO, the act is a collection of individual laws aimed specifically at combating the influence of organized crime in legitimate business. More specifically, RICO makes it *"unlawful to conduct or conspire to conduct an enterprise whose activities affect interstate commerce by committing or agreeing to commit a pattern of racketeering activity."*

Prior to RICO, law enforcement was limited to taking down individual mob bosses and racketeers. Unfortunately, this did little to thwart organized crime. Mob bosses and racketeers were all too quickly replaced. Furthermore, jailing a mob boss failed to disrupt the actual target of the government's efforts, i.e., the underlying criminal enterprise.

The passage of RICO changed everything. Drafted by

121

Professor G. Robert Blakely of the Notre Dame Law School, RICO allowed law enforcement to go after the entire criminal enterprise and, most importantly, its organization and money. Under RICO, a person or corporation found guilty can be fined up to $25,000 and sentenced to twenty years in prison for each count of racketeering *along with the forfeiture of all ill-gotten gains and interest in any business connected to those racketeering activities.*

Applying RICO in General:

While RICO was originally viewed as government's tool for prosecuting the Mafia and other forms of organized crime in the 1970s, it was always intended to have a far greater application. To quote Professor Blakely, *"We don't want one set of rules for people whose collars are blue or whose names end in vowels, and another set for those whose collars are white and have Ivy League diplomas."* Simply stated, Congress never intended RICO to just apply to the Mob. In fact, RICO has been a far more common response to white collar crime than the racketeering and Mob boss activities that are so popular with Hollywood.

In principle, RICO is simple to apply and extremely broad in scope. In fact, it was this simplicity, breadth and scope that made RICO such an effective tool for prosecuting the mob. However, the same can't be said for determining civil cases. Here, the simplicity of the act, along with its breadth and scope, encouraged attorneys to view RICO as an expedient way to drag legitimate businesses into court on all-too-thin claims of fraud and abuse. In fact, the practice became so prevalent that the U. S. Supreme Court was compelled to construct specific guidelines for determining the validity of civil suits filed under RICO. The Court also took steps to separate routine business practices from what can be considered a criminal enterprise.

From everything I can learn, this narrowing of RICO is responsible for the bulk of the frustration felt by a long list of capable attorneys who failed in their attempts to apply RICO to HMOs in the 1990s. While these attorneys were clearly convinced that HMOs were engaged in an enterprise designed to defraud enrollees for profit, it was and continues to be quite another matter to prove it in a court of law. Consider for a moment that some states, such as Pennsylvania, have legislatively empowered managed-care insurers to withhold payment whenever they believe a particular course of care is unjustified. Furthermore, even where such legislative authority does not exist, insurers have obtained state approval of their provider contracts, thus establishing their right to withhold payment in the same situation. In short, the states have sanctioned the very decisions plaintiffs want to attack. Consequently, insurers have every right to assert an affirmative defense in that: 1.) their denials of payment are a legally authorized business practice and 2.) the parties involved are simply fulfilling recognized roles in the market. And, given that the Supreme Court has ruled that a valid complaint under RICO requires a criminal enterprise of more than one party performing acts outside a legitimate role in the market, it should not be too surprising that these earlier attempts to apply RICO to HMOs and the managed-care insurance industry have essentially failed across the board. *"The strategy for vilifying HMOs and demonizing managed-care has failed."* (Consumers Versus Managed Care: The New Class Action, Clark C. Havighurst, Health Affairs, July 2001).

Why Past Attempts to Apply RICO Failed:

In order to establish a claim under RICO, a plaintiff must allege (1.) *conduct*, (2.) *of an "enterprise*," (3.) *through a pattern*, (4.) *of racketeering activity* (Lum v. Bank of Am., *361 F.3d* 217,223 3d Cir. 2004). Let's address each element in turn.

(1)   The Element of "Conduct":
One must have a factual basis for charging a defendant with the commission of one or more of some thirty-five federal and state crimes. Moreover, it's generally believed that there should be at least two identifiable crimes for a successful action.

(2)   The Existence of an "Enterprise":

One must allege and prove the existence of two distinct entities: a defendant (a person or corporation) and an "enterprise" that is not the same person by a different name. The RICO statute defines *enterprise* as "any individual, partnership, corporation, association or other legal entity, and any union or group of individuals associated in fact although not a legal entity. Moreover, in order to establish an enterprise, one must provide: proof of an ongoing organization, proof that the associates function as a continuing unit, and proof that the enterprise is an entity separate from the pattern of activity in which it engages.

(3)   Through A Pattern:

To show a pattern of racketeering activity, one must be able to show the existence of at least one of four specified relationships between the defendant(s) and the "enterprise": 1.) Either the defendant(s) invested the proceeds from the pattern of racketeering activity into the "enterprise"; or 2.) The defendant(s) acquired or maintained an interest in, or control over, the "enterprise" through the pattern of racketeering activity; or 3.) The defendant(s) conducted or participated in the affairs of the enterprise through the pattern of racketeering activity; or 4.) The defendant(s) conspired to do one or more of these three. In essence, one must be able to show that the "enterprise" is the illegal device of the racketeers. Furthermore, the U.S. Supreme Court has instructed federal courts that a *"pattern"* must *"have the same or similar purposes, results, participants, victims, or methods of commission or otherwise are interrelated by distinguishing characteristics and are not isolated events."* (H.J. Inc. v. Northwestern Bell Telephone Co.)

(4)   Racketeering Activity:

Here, one must be able to prove that at least one "activity" within the "pattern" of "enterprise" activity is a violation of state and/or federal law.

I hope that a reading of the above elements provides a fairly clear understanding of why earlier attempts to hold the managed-care insurance industry accountable under RICO failed. Plaintiffs were simply unable to show the existence of an "enterprise" other than an insurance company. Furthermore, the parties that plaintiffs attempted to include in an "enterprise" could be shown to be performing accepted roles in the normal course of business. Equally important has been the inability to prove the existence of a criminal act assignable to an "enterprise." Insurers are large, sophisticated companies with attorneys smart enough to avoid documenting any such policy or program, even if one existed. In addition, the economic incentives plaintiffs have cited were, at best, open to interpretation. But probably the most important factor in the failure of these attempts to sue insurers under RICO has been that the suits were seen by the courts as attempts to bring down the entire structure of employer-supplied managed-care health insurance authorized by Congress. Quoting again from Pegram, no *"HMO organization could survive without some incentive connecting physician reward with treatment* rationing" and *"the profit incentive to ration care"* goes *"to the very point of any HM* scheme." (U. S. Supreme Court Unanimous Decision in Pegram et al. v. Herdrich, 2000). I believe that all attorneys will readily acknowledge that the courts will do all they can to avoid invalidating an entire structure that both state and federal government have created. Once again quoting from Pegram, adopting the plaintiff's complaint *"would be nothing less than the elimination of the for-profit HMO."*

The question then becomes: Is there some other way to use RICO to hold the managed-care insurance industry accountable for what the U. S. Supreme Court has acknowledged is the denial of coverage and care at its very core?

In his book *Deadly Spin* and in his testimony before Congress,

Wendell Potter, a retired senior executive from the insurance industry and whistleblower, said, *"We have good reason to question the honesty and trustworthiness of the insurance industry"* and the PR of insurers " *is killing health care and deceiving Americans."* These are also widely held opinions of the American people. But how do we hold the managed-care insurance industry accountable for the fraudulent practices Wendell Potter addresses in his book and testimony? How do we make RICO work as it was intended to work? How do we make RICO work for average Americans who are being deceived, damaged, and in the case of Sandra Lobb, denied of life itself?

Charting a New Approach to RICO:

I am not about to claim I know how to succeed where so many have failed. I am not an attorney, and I am certainly no Robert Blakey. But what I can do is to propose a new RICO interpretation and test it against the Supreme Court's list of elements for determining a valid RICO complaint. Also, since RICO allows both prosecutions by a U.S. Attorney and civil suits by private parties damaged by a criminal enterprise, I will assume that the elements for a valid prosecution and a valid civil action are one and the same.

We begin our new approach to RICO where our first book, *The Great Health Care Fraud*, left off. We begin with: 1.) The misuse and misrepresentation of the state-mandated Enrollee Hold Harmless clause, 2.) The use of this clause to deny enrollees their right of contract, due process, liberty, and privacy in accessing needed health care, and 3.) The misrepresentation and fraud that insurers use in denying these rights. These three elements form the core of a new approach. For, rather than asking the courts to bring down an entire health care system that government has intentionally created, the new approach to RICO is centered on simply asking the courts whether <u>federal law allows this loss of an enrollee's right of contract, due process, liberty, and privacy in freely accessing needed health care.</u>

Rather than *"vilifying HMOs and demonizing managed care"*

as earlier RICO actions were accused of attempting to do, we would simply be asking the court whether a managed-care insurer should be allowed to: 1.) Use the all-too clear language of the Enrollee Hold Harmless clause to deny enrollees their right of contract, due process, liberty, and privacy in accessing needed health care, 2.) Hide their provider contracts along with its Enrollee Hold Harmless clause from enrollees, whom it most affects and 3.) Secretly use it to ration health care for the financial benefit of the insurer and its contracted "enterprise" of in-network doctors, hospitals, other health care providers, and the employers who purchase these managed-care plans. Therefore, we would not be asking the court to rule on whether an individual has a constitutional right to health care. We would not even be asking whether an insurer can ration health care and coverage. We would only be asking the court to rule on whether an enrollee has a right to access care without misrepresentation, fraud, and the unauthorized interference of an insurer in an enrollee's doctor-patient relationship. Or, stating it even more simply, we would not be asking whether an individual has a right to receive health care. **We would be asking whether an individual has a right to "*access*" health care at their own expense and outside the hidden and unauthorized interference of an insurance company, to which the individual owes no duty or obligation. And we would be asking it under the imposition of a federal mandate to purchase that very insurance, i.e., Obamacare.**

An equally strong argument for this new approach to RICO is that the moving party would be simply asking the federal courts to allow enrollees to exercise what the U. S. Supreme Court cited as the intent of Congress in its decision in Aetna v. Davila, dated June 21, 2004. Here the Supreme Court clearly stated that : "*Upon the denial of benefits, respondents could have paid for the treatment themselves and then sought reimbursement through a §502(a)(1)(B) action.*" And, "*Congress' intent to make the ERISA enforcement mechanism exclusive would be undermined if state causes of action . . . were permitted.*" And, "*The six carefully integrated civil enforcement provisions found in §502(a) of the statute as finally enacted . . . provide strong evidence that Congress did not intend to authorize other remedies that it simply forgot to incorporate expressly.*" Consequently, managed-care insurance companies' use of the Enrollee Hold Harmless clause to not only trespasses on an enrollee's doctor-patient relationship and right to access health care, but they very clearly substitute their own appeal process for the very specific remedy cited by the U. S. Supreme Court as the sole remedy intended by Congress.

Summarizing all this in my non-attorney way, the U. S. Supreme Court has ruled that the only recourse an enrollee can have, when wrongfully denied coverage, is to pay for the care and then sue to recover the cost under ERISA. However, to do that, a provider must accept the enrollee's payment, which a provider cannot do under the terms their provider contract and its Enrollee Hold Harmless clause. Consequently, it's the old "you can't get there from here" in spades. Since the provider can't accept an enrollee's payment, care can only be provided free of charge. And since there can be no payment, there will very likely be no rendering of care and certainly no cost of care. In addition, given no rendering of care and certainly no cost of care, there can be no basis for a suit under ERISA's *"reimbursement through a §502(a)(1)(B) action."* The insurer simply walks away a bit richer while an enrollee is left confused, untreated, and without any recourse other than the insurer's appeal process.

Any way one looks at it, it's a complete emasculation of what Congress and the Supreme Court have cited as the sole enforcement mechanism for a wrongful denial of coverage.

An important part of this new approach to RICO is the ability to position the states so that they have to either tacitly support the litigation or remain a nonparticipant in a purely federal matter. In other words, while I truly believe the states have been complicit in allowing insurers to exercise their unauthorized interference in the rights of an enrollee, I will argue that: 1.) They have had every right to interpret the Enrollee Hold Harmless clause (their legislation) as they have seen fit per rulings of the U.S. Supreme Court, 2.) They have done no more than support the intent of Congress, and 3.) Managed-care's use of the Enrollee Hold Harmless clause beyond the intent of the states has been within the bounds of state law. In other words, from the states' point of view, their house has remained in order and any issue of constitutionality or wrongful denial of coverage is purely a federal matter to be decided under applicable federal law. In essence, I'm betting that no state is about to go into federal court and risk having to acknowledge that they knowingly infringed the constitutional rights of enrollees to access health care at their own expense while deliberately misleading the enrollees in their state for more than twenty years. Far better to simply, as they say, throw the insurers under the bus and remain above the fray.

Once again my naiveté and non-attorney status is going to allow me to argue that this new approach is a virtual slam dunk. The mandate in Obamacare makes the issue a federal matter. The contract language of the Enrollee Hold Harmless clause speaks for itself. The insurance industry's use of its own interpretation of the language is well documented and easily proven. And, their efforts to keep their provider contracts and the Enrollee Hold Harmless clause secret as well as their misleading statements on coverage and rationing are readily available from a wide range of court records and documents. Furthermore, their criminal enterprise can be readily shown through the countless provider contracts and purchase agreements with doctors, hospitals, other health care providers and employers.

How can a federal court rule that an insurance company has the right to secretly deny an enrollee the right to contract, disclosure, process, liberty, and privacy in accessing health care when the U. S. Supreme Court has already ruled that a local sewer authority can't raise a citizen's sewer rate one dollar without providing both notice and process? Or a school can't suspend a child without providing notice and an opportunity to appeal the decision. They simply can't and remain consistent with the law and the Court's earlier rulings. And, need I say it once again? This is why The Heritage Foundation, conservatives and the Republican Party are so frightened by Obamacare and its mandate to acquire health insurance.

Applying the Required Elements to the New Approach:

In order to establish a claim under RICO, a plaintiff must allege (1) *conduct*, (2) *of an "enterprise*," (3) *through a pattern*, (4) *of racketeering activity* (Lum v. Bank of Am., *361 F.3d* 217,223 3d Cir. 2004). So we will address each element in turn. However, we will not bore all the non-attorneys with details that are best left to the knowledgeable lawyers who would litigate this new approach.

1. <u>Conduct</u>:

Managed-care insurance companies' unauthorized use of the Enrollee Hold Harmless clause to deny enrollees both coverage and access to health care while effectively barring them from the only recourse Congress and the U. S. Supreme Court allow for such loss.

2. <u>Of an Enterprise</u>:

The defendant is an insurance company that pursues the above conduct through an "Enterprise" comprised of contracted separate entities that are brought together under: 1.) the insurer's unauthorized use of the Enrollee Hold Harmless clause, 2.) the insurer's provider contracts and 3.) the insurer's other controlling documents, contracts, and certificates of insurance. Therefore, the "Enterprise" includes the insurance company, all in-network physicians, all in-network hospitals, all other in-network providers of skilled health care, and all contracted employers.

3. <u>Through a Pattern</u>:

Through a pattern of deliberate nondisclosure, misrepresentation, fraud, and intimidation, all under the umbrella of state action.

4. <u>Of Racketeering Activity Involving</u>:

a.) Fraud

b.) Extortion

c.) Mail and Wire Fraud

d.) Bank Fraud

e.) Breach of Fiduciary Duty Under ERISA

f.) Violation of The Hobbs Act, and

g.) A host of state consumer protection laws

5. <u>The Gain to Insurers and Damage to Enrollees</u>: The insurersConduct and Pattern of Racketeering Activity are all to the gain of a Defendant Insurance Company and the Enterprise it controls at the direct expense of Enrollees. The insurance company is allowed to: 1.) Enforce its decisions on rationing care outside the view of enrollees, 2.) Eliminate enrollees' only recourse as determined by Congress and the U. S. Supreme Court, 3.) Intimidate its in-network providers with a very real threat of nonpayment, 4.) Force providers to keep silent, 5.) Escape its ERISA responsibility to disclose its unauthorized interference in a doctor-patient relationship that enrollees are led to believe is their own, 6.) Reduce both what insurers pay for care and what employers pay for insurance, 7.) Lower its state-mandated reserve requirements, and 8.) Grow its profits. On the other hand, enrollees are: 1.) Secretly stripped of a doctor-patient relationship that they are led to believe they have, have every reason to believe they have, and must depend on for literally life itself; 2.) Secretly stripped of notice, process, contract, privacy, and liberty in accessing health care; 3.) Fraudulently billed by providers while ERISA fiduciaries (the insurer and the employer) stand silently aside, encouraging enrollees to believe it is their plan, their doctor, and *their bill.*

In Summary:

The above information is in no way meant to be a complete tutorial on a new approach to RICO. The subject is far too complicated for a book such as this and this author. What the chapter is meant to do is to disclose what the combination of the managed-care insurance industry's use of the Enrollee Hold Harmless clause and the Obamacare mandate can mean for RICO litigation.

These are: 1.) state-approved provider contracts with 2.) state-mandated language in the form of Enrollee Hold Harmless clause that 3.) cannot see changes to terms and conditions without first returning the contract to the state for approval, thus meeting the requirement of the Hobbs Act for "extorting" property/money by using the camouflage of legal authority. The property being taken by the "managed-care enterprise" being in the form of enrollees' doctor-patient relationship and the payments for health care that is illegally and fraudulently denied. Remember, even though an employee obtains health insurance as a benefit through his or her employer, the cost of that care is described as an integral part of the employee's compensation as well as his or her RICO protected benefit package. It just isn't counted as taxable income.

The following sections provide a brief overview of what this non-attorney sees as primary charges under a new approach to RICO. However, since there are countless state and federal laws and regulations that are applicable, the charges described below are far from a complete list. They are simply meant to provide examples of what could be charged under a new approach to RICO.

a.)　Extortion:

For the purposes of RICO, what we commonly think of as extortion is called a violation of the Hobbs Act (18 U.S.C. § 1951). In essence, the Hobbs Act elevates all but the simplest acts of robbery and extortion to the level of a federal crime chargeable under the RICO laws. More specifically, the Hobbs Act states:

*Whoever in any way or degree **obstructs**, delays, or affects* **commerce**, *or the movement of any article or* **commodity** *in commerce, by robbery or* **extortion** *or attempts or conspires so to do or commits or threatens physical violence to any person or property* **in furtherance of a plan** *or purpose to do anything in violation of this section shall be fined under this title or imprisoned for not more than twenty years, or both.*

As used in this section:

(1) The term robbery *means the wrongful taking or obtaining of personal property from the person or in the presence of another, against his will by means of actual or threatened force, or violence, or fear of injury, immediate or future, to his person or property, or property in his custody or possession, or the person or property of a relative or member of his family or of anyone in his company at the time of the taking or obtaining.*

(2) The term **extortion** *means the* **obtaining of property from another**, *with his consent, induced by the wrongful use of actual or threatened force, violence, or fear, or* **under the color of official right**.)

(3) The term **commerce** *means commerce within the District of Columbia, or any Territory or Possession of the United States, all commerce between any point in a State, Territory, Possession, or the District of Columbia and any point outside thereof, all commerce between points within the same State through any place outside such State and* **all commerce over which the United States has jurisdiction**.

The above bold type and underlining are, of course, not in the actual Act. I've chosen to highlight these portions of the text to identify what this non-attorney believes best supports the use of RICO in this instance. However, I could just as easily argue that the wrongful taking of an individual's doctor-patient relationship and the access it affords to necessary health care constitutes "robbery" under "fear" of injury from a loss of health insurance. The point is, that regardless of which course is chosen, the managed-care insurance industry wrongfully takes an enrollee's doctor-patient relationship and the access it provides to necessary health care as part of a carefully constructed "enterprise" that uses: 1.) fraud, 2.) "color of official right," and 3.) fear to achieve its ends.

b.)   Mail and Wire Fraud:

The most frequently used charge in RICO civil actions is the charge of mail and wire fraud. That is largely because the mail and wire fraud statutes essentially make it a crime for anyone to use the mail or wire services to commit a fraud. Furthermore, the fraudulent statements themselves do not have to be transmitted by mail or wire. The scheme to defraud simply has to be advanced, concealed, or furthered through the use of the mails or wires. And, because every business or enterprise uses the mail and wire services to conduct its operations, almost any business or enterprise that engages in fraud can be sued under RICO.

However, it's the sheer breadth of this application that has proven to be the greatest limitation in pursuing mail and wire fraud under RICO. And while these limits should not affect the use here, it does merit mentioning.

Perhaps the greatest limitation to converting a common law fraud into a RICO claim of mail and wire fraud is the aversion most federal courts have to RICO claims based solely on this alleged offense. See Sedima, S.P.R.L. v. Imrex Co., 473 U.S. 479, 500 (1985).

> *Underlying the Court of Appeals' [dismissal of the claim] was its distress at the "extraordinary, if not outrageous" uses to which civil RICO has been put. Instead of being used against mobsters and organized criminals, it has become a tool for everyday fraud cases brought against "respected and legitimate enterprises."*

And,

The "extraordinary" uses to which civil RICO [charges] have been put appear [to be] the result of the breadth of the predicate offenses, in particular the inclusion of wire [and] mail . . . fraud. . . .

Consequently, mail and wire fraud need to be seen as no more than a contributing element in a larger criminal "enterprise" of "extortion" stretching across a managed-care insurance company's many contracted participants.

c.)   Bank Fraud:
The RICO bank fraud statute is potentially every bit as broad as the mail and wire fraud statutes. Specifically, it states:

Whoever knowingly executes, or attempts to execute, a scheme or artifice:
1. *To defraud a financial institution, or*
2. *To obtain any of the moneys, funds, credits, assets, securities, or other property owned by, or under the custody or control of a financial institution, by means of false or fraudulent pretense, representation, or promises shall be fined not more than $1,000,000 or imprisoned for not more than 30 years, or both.* (18 U.S.C. § 1344)

Although most commonly viewed as a charge that requires some form of direct loss to a bank or financial institution, that simply isn't the case. Once again, the statute merely requires that the fraudulent enterprise uses banks or financial institutions to advance its scheme of fraud and/or extortion. Consequently, Bank Fraud arguably applies whenever a scheme to defraud enables the perpetrator (such as an insurer) to obtain any funds *"under the custody or control of"* a bank. In short, the bank fraud statute is violated whenever an employee authorizes the required monthly premium to be released to an insurance company. This is particularly true today when essentially every employee is required to make some level of direct contribution to his or her health insurance.

d.)   <u>Breach of ERISA Fiduciary Duty</u>:

I trust we can all agree that a managed-care health insurance company qualifies as a fiduciary under ERISA. After all, they are the designers of whatever plan an enrollee has and by the very nature of these plans have assigned themselves the role of "managing" an enrollee's health care expenses. Consequently, the failure of insurers to disclose the effect that their contractual Enrollee Hold Harmless clause has on an enrollee's doctor-patient relationship and freedom to access health care at their own expense can only be a direct and deliberate breach of their fiduciary duty under ERISA. In very simple English, the complete and sweeping efforts of insurers to keep their use of the Enrollee Hold Harmless clause secret and to systematically mislead enrollees on this issue constitute an outrageous abuse of fiduciary duty that is more consistent with the workings of the Mafia than a legitimate business entrusted with the lives of hundreds of millions of Americans.

To support this assertion, we need only return to what I cited earlier as Thomas and Beverly Dorr v. Sacred Heart Hospital, No. 98-1772, where the Wisconsin Court of Appeals ruled that the *"enrollee hold harmless provision of the Provider Agreement between the hospital and Group Health"* (the Dorrs' HMO) *"operate to exclude a debt owed the hospital by the Dorrs."* The court further affirmed the applicability of charges against the hospital for false representation, unfair debt collection practice, breach of contract, racketeering, tortious interference with a contract, and punitive damages. While this ruling involves a hospital, the court's findings are even more applicable to an insurance company that fails to disclose the impact of the Enrollee Hold Harmless clause and their provider contracts and systematically misleads enrollees about the effect they have on an enrollee's freedom to access the best available health care.

Summing Up This New Approach to RICO:

Where past efforts to use the RICO statute to hold managed-care insurers accountable for their rationing of "necessary and appropriate" health care have been largely ineffective, the individual mandate in Obamacare ushers in a whole new world. Because Obamacare requires each of us to acquire health insurance that effectively can only be a managed-care health plan that secretly strips us of our doctor-patient relationship, our right to access care at our own expense and our right to understand our medical bills, and does so through a network of state sanctioned but secret interlocking contracts, we are presented with a wide array of new approaches to RICO. In short, the individual mandate in Obamacare allows us to strip the rationing policies and practices of managed-care health insurers bare and stand them before a federal court to face the most basic of constitutional questions. Can such an insurer use a hidden contracted enterprise to strip enrollees of their doctor, their freedom to purchase needed health care and any and all due process? - - - I've yet to meet the attorney who believes they can!

....

TEN

"Every excuse I ever heard
made perfect sense to the
person who made it:"
Dr. Daniel T. Drubin

A New and Huge Liability for Employers

Employers have been extremely successful in convincing employees that the employer has no direct responsibility for the health insurance that they provide for their employees. Employers have simply stepped back and directed all questions and criticism to whatever insurance company provides the employer's plan. However, any reasonable analysis of ownership and responsibility creates a very different picture.

It should come as no surprise that health insurance is an extremely competitive market, particularly when it comes to large employers. The search for ever more cost-effective health plans has been a driving force behind changes in managed-care insurance for more than thirty years. In reality, employers own the vast majority of health insurance in the country and can be shown to be directly responsible for the steps that insurers have taken to make their plans more cost-effective — steps that the U. S. Supreme Court has ruled involve the rationing of health care as the *"very point"* of any managed-care health plan. But, even more to the point, how can a major employer with its stable of competent attorneys claim they don't understand the contracts they sign or the health plans they purchase for their employees? The truth is that they can't.

In a recent discussion I had over breakfast with a good friend and senior attorney at one of the country's largest companies, my attorney friend argued that there is no way his company could be expected to understand the details of the health plan they provide for their employees. In response, I begged him for the opportunity to contest his position in court. I pointed out that he would be asking the court to believe that his company, with its army of well-paid attorneys, is not capable of understanding the contracts they sign or the health plan they provide their employees. My attorney friend then laughed and surrendered his argument. The simple truth is that major employers cannot successfully argue that they don't understand the contracts they signed or the details of their health plans. They have just never been held accountable.

Once again, Obamacare changes everything. Once, the issue of the rationing and the managed-care industry's use of the Enrollee Hold Harmless clause bubbles to the surface, as it undoubtedly will, one of the most attractive targets for class action lawsuits will be large employers who have knowingly denied their employees their right of contract, process, liberty, and privacy in their ability to access health care in order to achieve a larger bottom line, i.e., a lower cost plan. Just ask yourself, how could a large employer argue that its choice of a health care plan wasn't driven by cost? My wife and I own a business, and I can assure you that each year, as the date for the renewal of our plan approaches, our insurer schedules a meeting with us to explain how they are changing our plan to minimize the growing cost of health care. It's an exercise that is absolutely necessary because our insurer knows his competition will be begging to be allowed to show us how their plan can save even more money.

Sure, the majority of employers want to provide their

employees with a credible plan, but the deciding factor in a competition between credible plans is cost, as it is with everything a business buys. Therefore, when you combine the drive of employers to cut the cost of their health plans with the reality that rationing is the "*very point*" of these plans, employers can be readily shown to have knowingly misrepresented their health plans for their own gain and at the direct expense of their naïve employees. In fact, all the charges I have described in the earlier parts of this book can be laid at the feet of large employers. They cannot claim to not know the details of their health plans because they have simply chosen to turn a blind eye to them. In short, they are sitting ducks for a knowledgeable attorney or employee who elects to hold them accountable for what ERISA makes an all-too clear fiduciary duty.

As with any suit, the seriousness of the threat is best measured by the damage one can lay at the feet of major employers. Here again there is just no place for an employer to hide. The scope and extent of the damage done to enrollees is enormous because it's not limited to flat denials of care. It includes all the lesser care and treatment that employees have received over the objections of what they were assured was their very own doctor. Furthermore, the loss dates back ten to twenty years. In addition, it includes all the fraudulent bills that insurers and providers have used for their own gain. And of course it will include punitive damages that the court will use to send a message that this form of conduct will not be tolerated.

As I have said repeatedly, I am not an attorney. However, I would love the opportunity to cross-examine a vice president of legal for a large employer that provides health insurance to its employees. I would love to watch this learned attorney attempt to explain how his company could be so naïve that they are not aware of: 1.) the contracts they have signed, 2.) the details of the health plan they have purchased, 3.) their responsibility under ERISA to inform enrollees of the details of the plan, 4.) the U. S. Supreme Court's decision in Pegram v. Hedrich, 5.) the part rationing plays in reducing the cost of their plan, and 6.) their full and sole ownership of their plan.

About a year or so ago I met with U. S. Congressman Joe Pitts (the Chairman of the House Subcommittee on Health) and Pennsylvania State Senator Dominic Pileggi (leader of the Pennsylvania Senate and a very competent attorney). In that meeting I described the liability Obamacare creates for large employers just as I have done above. Both of these gentlemen indicated their agreement with the points I am raising. However, after Congressman Pitts asked why I cared if enrollees aren't allowed to pay for their own health care, these two gentlemen had no place to go. Congressman Pitts had acknowledged that the Enrollee Hold Harmless clause secretly bars providers from getting paid unless they comply with the decisions of an insurance company, and neither man could defend it under our legal system. Neither man was able to refute my reply that they *"have no right to take it, let alone to take it secretly."*

Simply put, essentially everything I have written earlier in the book can be laid at the feet of an employer. Employers own the vast majority of health plans in the country and have a defined fiduciary obligation to manage these plans in a fully transparent manner and solely for the benefit of their enrollees. It's not only that simple, it's the law — federal law!

One Last but Important Point:

In preparing for the breakfast with my attorney friend that I describe above, I had given him a copy of the draft of this book to review and edit. So as we concluded our discussion of the material in the book, I asked him what he would do if he received a copy of the book at work via certified mail. His answer was almost immediate. He said *"Probably nothing."* I then reminded him that once he could be shown to have received the book and the material it contains, to do nothing would be to accept a personal liability for the charges cited in the book. I reminded him that as an attorney for his company he could not turn a blind eye to the hidden terms and conditions in his company's health plan without accepting personal liability for hiding these terms and conditions. My friend thought for just a moment and then said very thoughtfully, "*I would pass it on.*"

Our health care system is full of individuals who have a fiduciary duty to put the interests of enrollees above their own. Up to the release of this book, they have all been able to hide behind a wall of misrepresentation, deliberate fraud and hidden contractual terms and conditions. However, once this wall has been pulled down, these individuals will have no place to hide. And, nowhere is this more obvious than for responsible managers and attorneys at the nation's largest employers.

ELEVEN

....

*"A day without sun-
shine is like, you know,
night:"* Steve Martin

A Damning Comparison with Medicare

An Important Disclaimer:

A number of people who were kind enough to edit the initial draft of this chapter criticized it for appearing to promote the value of Medicare over private insurance. Let me make it crystal clear. There is absolutely no intent here to promote a single payer government system over free market private health insurance. No intent what so ever!

The purpose of this book has always been to simply disclose the truth about our private managed-care health insurance and to leave the ultimate design of a legally acceptable private health care system to others. Consequently, the purpose of this chapter is simply to show that the private managed-care insurance industry knows exactly what it is doing when it secretly strips enrollees of their doctor-patient relationship, their freedom to access health care at their own expense and any and all due process.

Just like the above quote from Steve Martin. When we compare the management of private managed-care health insurance with that of Medicare, the deliberate fraud in private managed-care health insurance becomes as painfully obvious as Mr. martin's sarcastic "*A day without sunshine is like, you know, night.*"

Same Structure and Control:

Created in 1965 and signed into law by President Johnson, Medicare made the financial burden of providing health insurance for retirees the responsibility of the federal government. In essence, Medicare was created to replace employer-supplied health insurance at age sixty-five. And, while this can be argued to be an oversimplification of more than thirty years of contentious battling over how to provide adequate health care for the nation's senior citizens, it's as far as we need go into what continues to be a hotly debated subject.

Congress had long supported employer-supplied health insurance as an alternative to a national single-payer system. However, this left open the question of how to provide insurance after an employee retired. Businesses weren't interested in shouldering that expense because seniors were known to need considerable care in their later years. Consequently, the government stepped in and created Medicare to replace employer-supplied managed-care health insurance following retirement. By so doing, Congress not only provided health insurance for aging retirees, but gave the market for employer-supplied private health insurance an added boost.

Since Medicare was created to replace employer-supplied health insurance, it should come as no surprise that it essentially mirrors what it was created to replace. In fact, Medicare not only has essentially the same design and structure as the private insurance it replaces, but it is administered by the very same organizations and people that administer private managed-care health insurance. The federal government simply contracts private insurers to administer Medicare. In fact, it's a huge source of revenue for these private insurers.

Like all private managed-care health insurance, Medicare is designed to: 1.) Operate through doctors, hospitals, and other health care providers that have contractually agreed to participate in the program, 2.) Provide coverage for "necessary and appropriate" care, 3.) Exclude coverage for only a few procedures or services, 4.) Require that providers bill only the insurer, and 5.) Effectively bar providers from billing a patient. Two programs, one private and one government. Both cut from essentially the same bolt of cloth.

While one might view these similarities as mere coincidence, I assure you they are not. They have serious legal implications. In both private managed-care insurance and Medicare, the in-network providers (all the approved doctors, hospitals, and suppliers of covered services) have agreed to provide "necessary and appropriate" care and be denied payment only when they fail to follow the procedures spelled out in the insurer's contract or the applicable regulations and law supporting Medicare. But most important, both private managed-care insurance and Medicare need to be able to determine "necessary and appropriate" care in order to control the cost of care — a determination the law specifically reserves for an attending physician.

While I have used the term "necessary and appropriate" to demonstrate the similarity between Medicare and private insurance, the actual term used by Medicare is *reasonable and necessary*. The 1965 Medicare legislation mandates the program not pay for items or services that are not *"reasonable and necessary."* However, I sincerely hope we can agree there is no practical difference between "necessary and appropriate" care and "reasonable and necessary" care. Both promise "necessary" care that can only be determined by an attending physician within the complexity of an individual case as a matter of law. And, both criteria attempt to find some means of incorporating cost in the determination of *"necessary"* care — a pursuit that neither Medicare nor private insurance has had much success when reviewed by the court. In fact, one federal appeals court has held that Medicare's attempts to incorporate cost in determining coverage are *"unambiguously closed."* Consequently, we will stay with "necessary and appropriate" for discussing what can only be identical criteria for coverage for both Medicare and private insurance. Necessary is necessary, and the attorneys for both forms of insurance face the same issues in attempting to moderate the determination of "necessary" based on cost.

This is not to imply that a provider's compensation (doctor, hospital or other health care provider) will be the same under both systems. Nor is this meant to imply that coverage will be the same for enrollees. Both are clearly not the case. In fact, this is a particularly large issue for doctors. I am simply making the point that the criteria for determining coverage are effectively the same for both forms of insurance.

The importance of these similar needs for determining "necessary and appropriate" care cannot be overstated as it is the nexus of both forms of insurance. Unfortunately, making their own determination of "necessary and appropriate" health care is a violation of law in every state in the country. As I have now repeated all too many times, only a properly licensed physician is authorized to determine "necessary and appropriate" health care and only when he or she has personally examined the patient. Obviously, both forms of insurance can't meet this requirement. Organizations, private or government, can't be licensed to practice medicine, and an insurer will never agree to examine a patient because of the liability it creates. Consequently, both forms of insurance (private and government) rely on the public's naivety and inability to separate the determination of "necessary and appropriate" care under law from the determination of "necessary and appropriate" care for insurance purposes. Once again, two forms of insurance, one private and one government, but both cut from the same bolt of cloth.

Similar but Oh-So Different:

It's within this need to determine "necessary and appropriate" health care that we find proof that the misrepresentation and fraud in private managed-care health insurance is both understood and deliberate. For, while Medicare reserves its determination of "necessary and appropriate" care until after care is rendered; private insurers require that the determination be made before any care is rendered. In essence, Medicare trusts attending physicians to deliver "necessary and appropriate" care and then makes payment and coverage an issue to be resolved solely between Medicare and the provider. Private insurers, on the other hand, demand attending physicians accept the insurer's determination of "necessary and appropriate" care before any care is rendered or lose all rights to bill either the insurer or the enrollee. In other words, while Medicare accepts attending physicians' determination of "necessary and appropriate" care, private insurers use their secret contracts to require attending physicians to either accept the insurer's decisions on "necessary and appropriate" care or provide the care free of charge. Furthermore, since private insurers are prohibited from determining "necessary and appropriate" care as a matter of law, they represent their decisions as a contractual determination of appropriate coverage rather than an infringement of an attending physician's legal authority and an enrollee's doctor-patient relationship.

These are huge differences. Under both private insurance and Medicare, a denial of coverage, which is simply a refusal to pay, can occur only when your doctor pursues something other than "necessary and appropriate" health care or the billing is mishandled. However, while Medicare allows your doctor to determine the care you need and render it, private insurers decide the care you will be allowed to receive and then bar payment for anything other than what they are willing to approve.

Furthermore, where Medicare goes to great lengths to properly assign the responsibility for appealing a refusal to pay, private insurers go to even greater lengths to improperly assign this responsibility. Quoting from a patient's copy of a May 10, 2013, Medicare Appeal Decision in a provider's Appeal of Non-payment, *"All Medicare providers are given instructions about services that are covered and not covered by the Medicare Program,"* and, *"Because of this, you* (the provider) *are held liable for the full charges for the services* (the services being appealed)," and, *"If the patient paid any money to you for the service at issue, Medicare will pay the patient back the amount that was paid to you."* Compare this with the extensive appeal procedures private insurers have established to make any appeal of coverage the *responsibility of the enrollee.* In fact, private insurance plans typically state that an enrollee's failure to properly appeal a denial of coverage forfeits the right to appeal.

Stating it as simply as I can, Medicare ensures its enrollees get the care prescribed by their doctor and then makes the appeal of any *denial of "coverage"* the responsibility of the provider. Private managed-care insurance, on the other hand, *denies "care"* and then directs any appeal of the denial: 1.) Onto the enrollee, 2.) Away from the insurer's provider contract, and 3.) Onto an insurance plan in which the enrollee is neither an owner nor a signatory. It's deliberate misrepresentation and fraud at its very worst.

However, if these very different approaches to determining coverage were no more than the product of two separate organizations, one might argue that there is little proof of any wrongdoing. However that is not the case. The two forms of insurance are administered by the very same people. The government simply contracts private insurance companies to administer Medicare. So, we have the very same people or organizations determining appropriate coverage for both forms of insurance.

Once again, these are huge differences that go to the very heart of the obligation for good faith and fair dealing, consumer fraud, our constitutional right to contract and process in accessing "necessary and appropriate" health care as well as the ERISA requirement for a clear and accurate description of an employer's health plan. Where Medicare pursues legal clarity and carefully avoids any direct interference with the doctor-patient relationship, private managed-care insurance does just the opposite — *and they do it in secret.*

Under Medicare, physicians are free to prescribe and render the "necessary and appropriate" care required by the nation's health care laws, their duty to the patient, and the physician's code of ethics. The only issue allowed is the question of who should pay for this "necessary and appropriate" care. So long as the procedure is not specifically excluded by Medicare and the physician provides the necessary documentation, Medicare pays for the care. If, for any reason, the physician or other provider suspects Medicare may not agree to pay for the care they are providing, they need only complete an Advance Beneficiary Notice of Noncoverage (Form CMS-R-131) to guarantee an enforceable bill. See Appendix 10.

Accordingly, under Medicare, a patient's doctor-patient relationship can be argued to remain intact because: 1.) The physician has agreed to treat patients within the Medicare system, 2.) The obligation this creates can be understood because it's defined in the law, and 3.) The physician is assured of payment so long as he or she provides the required documentation. And, while the contentious issues of appropriate compensation and burdensome documentation for a participating physician are very real, they reside within the Medicare system and arguably outside an enrollee's doctor-patient relationship.

Private managed-care health insurance can make no such claim. Consider once again how a hospital is likely to react to attempts by your doctor to get the care he or she believes you need and your private insurer is refusing to approve. Under the law, so long as your doctor prescribes the care and there is an offer to pay for it, the hospital has to provide it. And, remember, everyone signs an agreement to pay for whatever their insurer fails to cover when they are admitted to a hospital. So the hospital already has your signed offer to pay along with your doctor's valid prescription for the care you need. However, the hospital knows it can't bill you for anything the insurer is refusing to cover. Consequently, the hospital knows it can't get paid for the care your doctor is prescribing. Furthermore, this unrecoverable cost is likely to be in the tens of thousands of dollars, if not more. And, once a hospital begins a course of treatment, the laws in every state require it to continue treatment so long as the patient requires the care. The only way out of this quagmire for the hospital is to get your doctor to change his or her mind and accept your insurer's decision on the care you should be allowed to receive.

While your doctor may have the best professional ethics, no

doctor can knowingly cost a hospital this kind of money and stay in its good graces. This is the hammer that private insurers hold over the head of an enrollee's doctor. It's also the seat of power for rationing health care in private managed-care health insurance. And, it's why I stated at the very start of this book that America's doctors are as much hostages to private managed-care health insurance as the enrollees they treat.

In short, how anyone can view the difference between Medicare and private managed-care health insurance as anything but proof of the deliberate severing of the doctor-patient relationship by private managed-care companies is beyond me. These are two forms of insurance administered by the same people. So when the same organizations that administer Medicare, with its protections of the doctor-patient relationship, turn around and <u>secretly</u> infringe an enrollee's doctor-patient relationship in order to ration health care in private managed-care insurance, there can be nothing less than the knowing and deliberate severing of the doctor-patient relationship. And for those who need further proof, you need only look at how private insurers direct a denial of coverage away from their provider contracts and onto a mythical insurance policy that enrollees do not and cannot own.

Yes, Medicare is a highly complex and regulated program, and yes, the role of government in health care deserves to be hotly debated. Even so, when measured solely in terms of its approach to preserving the duty a physician owes to his or her patients, Medicare can serve to shine a bright light on the deliberate misrepresentation and fraud embodied in private managed-care health insurance.

Medicare may be a lot of things to different people, and it is far from a perfect system, but it provides us with an excellent example of how government has worked to preserve the essence of the doctor-patient relationship while private insurance has conspired to do just the opposite.

Why So Different?

Given the animosity many of us have for private insurance

companies, it's easy to blame their infringement of the doctor-patient relationship on a pursuit of power and ever greater profits. Easy, but almost certainly not the case. It's far more likely a product of the difference between what the government can do and the constraints the law places on private insurance.

Certainly, both Medicare and private insurance have a similar need to control costs. Medicare needs to operate within a budget established by Congress. Private insurance companies need to operate within a budget that delivers the growth and profits their shareholders and the market demand. What's more, both forms of insurance face the same two primary areas of cost control: 1.) The price they pay for care, and 2.) The nature of the care determined to be "necessary and appropriate," i.e., the type of care they have to pay for.

The first of these two areas of cost control is extremely contentious because it involves the compensation that providers receive for their services. However, it's also the easiest to manage. Medicare and the private insurers simply use their all-too-heavy hand to drive down the price they pay for care. The second area of cost control presents a far greater challenge for both forms of insurance.

To understand this challenge and why Medicare and private insurers approach it differently, we first need to agree that Medicare is not insurance. It's simply a government program designed to pay participating health care providers for products and services in accordance with criteria defined in the law. As such, Medicare is really no different from any other government program that offers payments based on a set of criteria established in the law. It is no more insurance than the federal government's food stamp program or the city of New York's program for housing assistance. And, since Medicare is simply a federal program to dispense payments, it lacks any and all authority to regulate the doctor-patient relationship without trespassing on the right of the states to regulate insurance and health care. As a result, Medicare has only one choice for controlling the nature of the care they have to pay for. This is the same means of control used by every form of government — constructing a mountain of specific reporting requirements that limit their obligation to pay for care. In short, they leave the determination of "necessary and appropriate" care to the attending physician, but make the payment for care contingent on all the required documentation being complete, timely, and accurate. It's a burdensome and inefficient program for participating physicians and providers, but it's really the only means Medicare has for controlling the nature of the care they have to pay for.

Private insurance is a completely different matter. Because private insurers are private businesses, they can't establish rules and regulations in the law that limit the care they have to pay for. Private insurers can only inject themselves into the doctor-patient relationship in order to limit what they have to pay for. They need a way to force physicians to accept their insurer's determination of "necessary and appropriate" care in order to control their costs and grow their profits.

In summary, because Medicare avoids infringing the doctor-patient relationship, it can be fully transparent in administering coverage. However, because private managed-care health insurance must infringe the doctor-patient relationship in order to control its costs and grow its profits, it has no choice but to hide the details of its health plans through carefully constructed misrepresentation and fraud.

In Summary:

Nothing I have said should be interpreted as an endorsement of Medicare or a national single payer system to replace private managed-care health insurance. Both systems have deep structural problems. And, both systems ration health care in order to control costs. However, Medicare is uniquely transparent in its dealings because the laws that govern the coverage it provides are available for anyone who chooses to read them. Private insurers provide no such transparency, nor can they afford to. Their provider contracts are not only hidden from enrollees and the public, but are deliberately misrepresented in order to provide direct control over the doctors and hospitals that we look to for health care and life itself.

When you have one group of people administering two very different approaches to transparency, the doctor-patient relationship and coverage, as we do in Medicare and private managed-care health insurance, there has to be a clear and well thought-out reason. The differences are just too big and consequential to be anything other than deliberate. Therefore, we can say with confidence that we have one group of managers who know exactly what private managed-care health insurance is doing to secretly and illegally infringe enrollees' doctor-patient relationship, access to care at their own expense and constitutional right to notice and process.

TWELVE

···

Your individual needs must "__capitulate__
to the needs of the community:"
                    Mark Bertolini, CEO of Aetna

The Future Managed-Care Wants

Some Background:

Unfortunately, the future we are being herded toward is becoming all too obvious. It's all around us. Doctors who are no longer our own personal physician, mega-hospitals that direct us in and out like an assembly line in a factory, and billing procedures so confusing that a Certified Public Accountant can't determine whether a bill is accurate. And it's all designed to hide a fundamental element in the American health care system — the rationing of health care for the profit of private enterprise and control of the government's cost of health care. It's a manipulation of the law and our values that is being so carefully hidden that even our finest journalists appear ignorant of the issue and its heavy cost to our American way of life.

The simple truth is that the rationing of health care is an everyday reality in the United States. In fact, countless readers of the U. S. Supreme Court decision in Pegram v. Hedrich have characterized it as a call for the American people to wake up to the existence of rationing as a fundamental element in managed-care health insurance. However, the insurance industry, our government, and most particularly the Republican Party refuse to acknowledge what the Supreme Court found so obvious. Instead, they, including the Democratic Party, would rather turn a blind eye to the existence of rationing along with the shredding of the Constitution and the violation of numerous federal and state laws that it creates. In short, they would rather protect the financial interests of big business than recognize the right of the individual American to access health care absent the illegal interference of a health care insurance company and big money.

In the March 4, 2013, edition of *Time* magazine, Steven Brill did a masterful job of describing the effect that big money has on our health care system. According to Brill, it has become *"a uniquely American gold rush — from Stanford, Conn., to Marlton, N.J., to Oklahoma City . . . ."* Brill goes on to report that *"the American health care market has transformed tax-exempt nonprofit hospitals into the town's most profitable business and largest employers, often presided over by the region's most richly compensated executives."* *The New York Times*, in a lead article on May 18, 2013, provides us with another excellent example of this transformation. In 2007 the Bayonne Medical Center was a bankrupt hospital in *"a faded blue-collar town 11 miles from Midtown Manhattan."* Today that same hospital charges the highest rates in the country and its profits have *"soared."*

But we don't have to rely on the words of reporters; we can readily see the same thing that drove Steven Brill to write his article for *Time* magazine. While visiting Houston, Mr. Brill noticed a group of glass skyscrapers lighting up the evening sky. *"The scene looked like Dubai,"* reports Brill. It was, in fact, the Texas Medical Center with 280 buildings sitting on nearly 1,300 acres. It's one of Houston's largest employers. I had the same experience while attending a conference at the University of Pennsylvania Medical Center. Stretching out over untold blocks of downtown Philadelphia and boasting the most modern and expensive construction, the size and grandeur of the facility is amazing. In fact, it screams money and power.

This is just the obvious part of what has become the single most dominant part of our national economy. Representing roughly twenty percent of our GDP, the health care industry will generate just under three trillion dollars of revenue in the coming year. That's trillion with a "t." And to insure this flood of money continues, the health care industry has spent $5.36 billion since 1998 on lobbying Congress. This dwarfs the $1.53 billion spent by the defense and aerospace industries and the $1.3 billion spent by oil and gas interests over the same period of time. In essence, the health care industry is committed to ensuring they keep the flood of money pouring in. However, because change is inevitable, particularly given the unacceptable rise in the cost of health care, the corporate leaders in our health care system are doing more with their billions of dollars than simply lobbying to maintain the status quo. They are working for a future that will accept change, but preserve their power and to control what is an ever-growing torrent of money. In short, they have a plan that not only preserves the role of managed-care in our health care system, but expands their authority to control it.

From the Horse's Mouth:

Fortunately, we don't have to guess at where it's all headed. Mark Bertolini, CEO of Aetna, took all the guesswork out of the issue in an in-depth interview he gave to Dylan Scott for the May 2013 issue of *Governing* magazine (see "The Future of Insurance in an Era of Health-Care Reform" at www.governing.com). In fact, Mr. Bertolini was so clear and unambiguous that one can only conclude that he believes that Aetna and the rest of the large players in the health care insurance industry have the future (our future) well in hand.

To provide some context for Mr. Bertolini's comments, Aetna has more than forty million enrollees, one million providers under contract, and yearly revenue of more than thirty billion dollars.

Furthermore, the future of this 160-year-old company depends on its ability to not just maintain its position in the health care market, but to grow its power and profits some three to five percent a year for as far as the eye can see.

The key to understanding Mr. Bertolini's and Aetna's plans for our future is his insistence that our future health care system must be built around what he calls *"population health management."* He describes it as a way to *"improve the health of the population in a way that provides a more valuable input into the economy of the country. So it would be an investment in productivity."* Mr. Bertolini goes on to say that Population Health Management *"would have a community based-organization that would not only be a large employer in the economy but also a key provider of economic input."* and that our health system would be *"a true popular health system . . . which would meet with the community and understand the ongoing demography, disease burden and trends."* It's a system where one's individual need for care *"would **capitulate** to the needs of that community over time."* He added that *"the outcome that we would measure* is" whether the *"economy is better off."*

Mr. Bertolini further explained that he and Aetna, along with the other large insurers, have: 1.) All the data necessary to understand *"how the system should be constructed,"* 2.) The *"technology"* to collect this necessary *"information"* on enrollees, and 3.) The *'financing capability to make sure that the investment is well handled."* It's a system where the American people would *"think of an insurance company . . . as a highly specialized bank"* that provides *"financing, risk management, reinsurance coverage . . . intellectual property, data and technology as the intelligence side of a health-care system."*

Most telling was Mr. Bertolini's answer to Dylan Scott's question of *"Are you doing this somewhere?* He said yes, *"in China."* Mr. Bertolini went on to say that Aetna will be working with the Chinese government *"to set up this type system"* because they *"don't have the barriers there that we have here."* The Chinese, he added, *"don't have entrenched interests . . . to overcome."* And

Aetna believes it can *"create a cresting wave phenomenon . . . that will allow us to try it here in the United States."*

And, as to what Mr. Bertolini forecasts for our doctors and hospitals, he was equally open and explicit. The new system will *"require us to go about our work differently. It's not a negotiation with providers over what to pay them, but a partnership with providers to understand what we're investing in and how we can both work together to make sure that investment achieves the maximum return."* And, *"**It really requires the providers to trust us in ways that they've never had to trust us**."*

Disconnected by Power and Money:

Surely Mr. Bertolini means exactly what he describes in his interview with Dylan Scott. His choice of words is far too specific to be anything other than a carefully tailored message designed to be more acceptable than the simple language of "We will be taking control of the nation's health care system, and the needs of individual enrollees will have to take a backseat to the financial needs of Aetna and the country." Instead, Mr. Bertolini's carefully crafted comments are clearly the product of a high-priced marketing team charged with sliding a very distasteful message past an all-too trusting and naïve American public.

Unlike Mr. Bertolini, I am more than willing to use plain English to express my equally clear and unambiguous response to his and Aetna's plans for our future. Let me say it as clearly as I can: "No F---ing way!" Furthermore, my Republican Party and its conservative wing should be just as clear in refuting Mr. Bertolini's plan. Because what he describes as *"barriers"* to his plan for a new health care system is what we commonly refer to as the U. S. Constitution, along with the word and spirit of state and federal law. Unlike China, where the only individual right to care that I am aware of is the right to a speedy execution if you upset the government, this country is grounded in the inalienable rights of the individual — rights that emanate from God and not government — rights that cannot be cast aside or ignored for the convenience and profit of a managed-care insurance industry or the perceived needs of government.

No, Mr. Bertolini, you can't trash the U. S. Constitution and the inviolable rights that we have fought and died for. You can't trash these rights any more than you, Aetna, and the rest of the insurance industry can sever the doctor-patient relationship through misrepresentation, hidden provider contracts, and slick wording designed to hide the details of your plans. The doctor-patient relationship predates this country and is one that, in terms of contract and the right to process, liberty, and privacy in accessing health care, cannot be simply trampled into the dustbin of history. Not unless you rewrite the Constitution and restructure more state and federal laws than I can count.

No, Mr. Bertolini, you can't simply ignore the rights of the individual as your carefully worded message proposes. Not once in your lengthy interview do you mention the rights and needs of the individual enrollee who is your ultimate customer. You speak only of collective needs for the economy, population management, the needs of the community, the need to ensure maximum return on investment and the need for our doctors to trust your decisions in ways they have never had to in the past. In fact, nothing can be more telling than the complete absence of any reference or consideration of the rights and needs of the individual enrollee. Instead, you make it all too clear that your industry's focus is solely on limiting access to health care for what you claim is the greater good and, of course, Aetna's profitability.

No Mr. Bertolini, you can't simply wipe away this nation's guarantee of individual rights and freedom through slick marking, misrepresentation and obfuscation. You can't recast a nation of individuals into a commune or peoples' republic by simply getting creative in how you and your industry structure and market your managed-care health plans.

However:

Unfortunately, what I have said Mr. Bertolini cannot do

is exactly what he, Aetna, and the entire managed-care insurance industry have been working toward for the past thirty-some years. In fact, they have laid siege to the doctor-patient relationship with a patience and focus best associated with the Chinese. The truth is that since the 1970s, Mr. Bertolini, Aetna, and the other powers in the managed-care insurance industry have steadily increased their control over the doctors and hospitals we look to for health care. Yes, the insurance industry hit a bump in the road in the 1990s with the HMO backlash. But they modified their provider contracts, adjusted health plans, and got Congress and the U.S. Supreme Court to eliminate any enrollee recourse outside of ERISA. The result has been that they have emerged stronger than ever and with the exact the same goal — to obtain ever greater power over what doctors and hospitals can provide in the way of covered health care.

The candor in Mr. Bertolini's comments has to be seen as a measure of his confidence in the managed-care industry's quest for control. Having maximized the control that can be obtained through their hidden provider contracts and Enrollee Hold Harmless clause, insurers are now pursuing an even greater level of control. Through direct acquisitions, mergers, and contractual affiliations, the insurance industry is making the American physician (your doctor and mine) either a direct employee or, in one form or another, a contract employee of the insurance industry. In fact, it's the only way the insurance industry can fulfill Mr. Bertolini's stated goal of having *"providers trust us in ways that they've never had to trust us."* Or in my more plain English, it's the only way that insurers can achieve the final say in the care enrollees will be allowed to receive — even if they are willing to use their own money to pay for the care they need and want.

Returning to the words of Mr. Bertolini in his interview with Dylan Scott, *"If you were to talk to my counterparts in the big companies, they would give you their version of what they're doing relative to changing the nature of relationships with providers. Some of them are buying practices and health systems. Others are trying to build collaborative relationships with them."* Once again he is plainly saying that the managed-care insurance industry is focused on gaining direct control over America's physicians. Slightly different approaches, but with a single outcome. It's an outcome designed to not only sever your doctor-patient relationship through secret provider contracts with an Enrollee Hold Harmless clause, but to gain complete control over your doctor by making your doctor an employee of the insurance industry. In essence, insurers get the power to ration care as they see fit and your doctor can only follow the instructions of the insurer — to *"trust us in ways that they've never had to trust us."*

Take my own family doctor, for example. He has been my doctor for more than thirty years. However, a few years back he sold his practice to a regional hospital that is owned by a large corporate health care chain. Since I had discussed my first book with him, I asked if being an employee, rather than an independent practitioner, has changed how he has to practice medicine. His answer was *"Absolutely yes!"* He explained that there are now clearly defined policies on what he can and cannot prescribe.

The really frightening part of all this is that what the insurance industry is doing is completely legal. Furthermore, the U. S. Supreme Court has ruled that doctors employed by a managed-care insurance company are not subject to the duty of care and liability assigned to an independent practitioner (Pegram v. Herdrich). This carries the clear implication that, in spite of my *"No F---ing Way,"* the insurance industry believes they have a smooth and open road to the future they want. Or at least they did up until the passage of Obamacare with its individual mandate.

So while I believe we all owe Mr. Bertolini a debt of gratitude for his candor in explaining where the insurance industry is headed, the brazenness of his comments is absolutely astounding. It's a brazenness that I can only associate with an accumulation of money and power that perverts one's sense of law, ethics, and responsibility — a feeling of being immune from the norms the rest of us live by.

That being said, I hope we can all agree that Mr. Bertolini's comments not only describe where the insurance industry is headed, but provides clear support for the issues I raise in this book. At the very least, his comments should eliminate any doubt that the insurance industry is determined to appropriate the authority of the American physician to determine the care an enrollee needs and will be allowed to receive. Or stated more simply, to openly ration the care you and I can receive even at our own expense. After all, Mr. Bertolini and his like heads of the managed-care insurance industry are headed for a system that: 1.) requires doctors to *"trust us in ways that they've never had to trust us,"* 2.) " **_capitulates_** *to the needs of the community,"* and *3.)* asserts that *"the outcome that we would measure is"* whether the *"economy is better off."* In my mind, it's a system deserving of the title from the World War II book, *"They Were Expendable."* The "They" being you, me and our loved ones when we are seen as costing the *"community,"* the *"economy"* or the insurer too much.

Their Only Competition:

It should be obvious that nothing can match the size and power of the insurance industry in our health care system. However, a recent change in the market has created a challenge to that size and power. Fully documented by Steven Brill in the March 4, 2013 edition of *Time* magazine, the nation has seen an explosion in the size of hospitals and other provider organizations. Driven by a need to counter the suffocating power of insurance companies and the outstanding opportunity for investment in the health care market, the number of acquisitions, mergers and contractual relationships within the health care market has changed the provider landscape. Hospitals are no longer a single institution. They are now far more likely to be but one hospital in a large corporate shell structured to dominate hospital services in a particular area of the country.

These new mega-hospitals can stand toe to toe with insurers when it comes to negotiating acceptable pricing. It's one of their most significant strengths. However, these mega-hospitals have the same need to control what doctors prescribe as the insurance industry. Because mega-hospitals must still look to insurers for payment, and insurers can retroactively deny such payment, mega-hospitals have to control what doctors prescribe if they are to control their costs. Thus, we are witnessing two large and powerful corporate entities battling for the same thing — control over the nation's doctors.

Nowhere has this battle been more evident than in Pittsburg, Pennsylvania. Here, Highmark Blue Cross and the University of Pittsburgh Medical Center (UPMC) have created a Gordian knot that the best minds in the State have been unable to resolve. Simply stated, Highmark Blue Cross controls the overwhelming majority of health insurance in the Pittsburgh area. UPMC controls the overwhelming majority of health services in the Pittsburgh area. In short, without a contract between these two corporate giants, the inhabitants of the Pittsburgh area can't use their Highmark managed-care insurance. Unfortunately, that contract expired on June 30, 2012.

The resulting impasse between Highmark and UPMC began when Highmark announced its intention to purchase five struggling hospitals in the Pittsburgh area. *"Having announced its intention to compete with UPMC as a producer, there cannot be any reasonable prospect for a contract renewal between Highmark and UPMC,"* UPMC spokesman Paul Wood. Mr. Wood was simply stating the obvious. UMPC can't remain financially viable if Highmark is allowed to establish direct control over a major portion of the area's doctors. On the other hand, the intransigent response of Highmark provides an excellent example of just how serious Highmark is in pursuing control of physicians in the Pittsburgh area.

The bad news for the residents of Pittsburgh is that regardless of who wins this struggle, it can only lead to higher costs for both health care services and insurance. And the really bad news for UPMC is that the State of Pennsylvania is not about to allow UPMC to win and effectively invalidate the existing health insurance for the entire Pittsburgh area. So, while the State can't force UPMC to sign a new contract with Highmark, it can and has extended the old contract until such time as UPMC agrees to negotiate a new contract with Highmark.

The bottom line is that while the new mega-hospitals are

likely to provide increasing competition for the control of the nation's doctors, this competition is not likely to weaken the stranglehold that the insurance industry has on our health care system. After all, the insurers supply the bulk of the money that hospitals and the entire health care system require. And as is always the case, money is the real seat of power.

In Summary:

We know where the managed-care insurance industry is headed. Their plans for the future are but an extension of the policies and practices they have been pursuing since the 1970s. Furthermore, if there was any doubt about their plans, Mr. Bertolini's candor strips it all away. In the simplest of terms, Mr. Bertolini, Aetna and the managed-care insurance industry see themselves well on the way to expanding their hidden power to ration health care in a system so intrusive and counter to our individual rights that it can only be tested in China — a system where the needs of the individual "*capitulates to the needs of the community*" — a system where they can force doctors (your doctor and my doctor) to trust insurers "***in ways that they've never had to trust***" insurers.

Very much like the focus and patience we have seen from China in capturing U.S. manufacturing, the managed-care insurance industry is committed to invading our right to access health care until the industry's control is so complete that it can't be undone. And, they will be hiding behind the country's growing need to control the cost of health care. In that way, they can remain absolutely confident that Washington will be in full support of their unprecedented power-grab.

The frightening part is that as farfetched and Orwellian as all this may sound, the history of health care and the staggering amount of money involved make the fulfillment of Mr. Bertolini's plans all too likely. For as the old saying goes, "*When money speaks, truth is silent.*"

The amount of money involved in health care along with the nation's preference for a private market solution virtually assures managed care insurance companies will continue to have a leadership role in our health care system. After all, they provide the overwhelming source of funding for health care and even administer the government's portion of health care funding. In short, Mr. Bertolini, Aetna, and the rest of the managed-care insurance industry can rest comfortably in the knowledge that they control the system and will continue to do so. The only question that remains is what we as a free people and a nation of laws will allow them to do in the name of administrating "our" health care.

I purposely left off the word *system* at the end of the last sentence because it is not the system that is at issue or so terribly wrong with where the insurance industry is headed. Under our capitalistic system, insurers can pretty much market whatever they choose. We not only allow it, we encourage it as a primary engine of growth for the economy. However, an insurer's freedom to market a product cannot void an individual's constitutional right to freely *access* the advice of his or her "doctor" and the care they and their doctor believe is "necessary and appropriate." These are absolutes in our system of laws. They are also absolutes that the insurance industry cannot change. And, they are absolutes that Mr. Bertolini, Aetna, the insurance industry, and their formidable army of attorneys fully understand. Consequently, it is these absolutes that insurance industry must circumvent. After all, the right of an individual to the advice and care of his or her doctor is anathema to rationing and, rationing is an essential part of every managed-care insurance plan and product.

THIRTEEN

....

Whatever is my right as a man is also
the right of another; and it becomes my
duty to guarantee as well as to possess:
Thomas Paine, Rights of Man

No Need to Play by Their Rules

Getting Care & Coverage Every Time:

While thwarting an insurer's interference in your doctor-patient relationship is really quite simple, the solution didn't come quickly or easily to me. It took years of litigation and study to discover a hole in the armor that managed care has created around their in-network physicians. In fact, my understanding arrived more like a flash of light from out of the blue than a product of reasoned analysis. That was largely because the insurance industry, with the help of the states, have made the terms and conditions used in managed-care health insurance deliberately misleading and false. Furthermore, who would ever believe a state would allow an insurer to prevent an enrollee from paying for their own health care?

Throughout my ten years of litigation I had thought of nothing but how to prove that we had been denied the right to pay for Sandy's care. I was consumed by it and my anger over her needless death. In short, my pursuit of justice became an obsession. And it was this obsession, along with my strong belief that our insurer had acted outside the law that kept me charging down a proverbial blind rabbit hole. I was immersed in the belief that any reasonable person could see that we had been denied the right to pay for Sandy's care.

While I am not the most outwardly religious man, I have always believed that God and fortune have been particularly kind to me. And once again, such was the case here. It was the end of the very last hearing that I would have in our pursuit of justice. The lead attorney for the insurer simply chose to take me aside to explain that we needed to withdraw our suit or face serious financial consequences. Not that he threatened me in any way. He simply explained the consequences of further litigation. That explanation moved on to a discussion of the Enrollee Hold Harmless clause and Ka-POW, I had my blinding flash of light. For the first time I was able to set my biases aside and connect the dots. I had my answer.

I can remember almost laughing as I told him that I finally understood what they were doing with their provider contracts. I said that the key to accessing care isn't being allowed to pay for it. **It's demanding the "right" to pay for it and the "access" this affords an enrollee under both the law and an insurer's provider contract**. I then gave him the following example. I should probably mention that the attorney I was speaking to was a very gracious black gentleman.

When a black American walks into a restaurant in the Deep South, he can be confident of getting a meal because the law requires the restaurant to serve him as long as he is willing to pay for the meal and the restaurant is capable of serving it. However, when he finishes his meal, the law says nothing about the restaurant having to bill him or to accept his money. The restaurant is completely free to provide the meal free of charge. They just have to provide the meal. Furthermore, if the restaurant has a sign over the front door stating "All Meals Free to Celebrate Our Grand Opening," the restaurant can't accept his money as a matter of law.

I then provided the attorney with an equivalent example in health care. If a properly licensed doctor prescribes care and the patient demonstrates a willingness to pay for the care, the hospital must supply it so long as it is an available service of the hospital. However, if the hospital has been so foolish as to have contracted away its right to bill the patient, that's the hospital's problem, not the patient's. The hospital has to provide the care free of charge. That's the law in every state in the country.

The look on the attorney's face was priceless. I have to believe that, like me, he had never stepped out of the box to view their well-constructed barriers to accessing care from the back side — to access coverage through the "*backdoor*" rather than through the front door that insurers control. It's a huge hole in their carefully constructed armor. It's also one that they can't close without completely restructuring the design of managed-care health insurance, i.e., your plan and mine.

But, let's go back to my restaurant example to be certain we all understand exactly what I am saying. The black American's right to receive a meal comes from the law's requirement that licensed restaurants must serve whoever enters, requests a meal, and is willing to pay for it — period! Now let's say the restaurant hangs a sign on the front door offering free food as part of a one-day promotion. Is the restaurant now free to deny people service? No way! The law requiring the restaurant to serve all customers equally is unaffected by the restaurant's billing decision. Therefore, so long as a customer enters the restaurant and is willing to pay, the restaurant has to serve him. However, when the customer goes to leave, a separate provision of the law bars the restaurant from billing the customer so long as the sign promising free food remains on the door.

Our nation's laws on health care and insurance have the same structure as my restaurant example. State health care laws and operating licenses require hospitals to provide care to everyone offering to pay for it so long as the care is prescribed by a properly licensed physician and within the hospital's capability. However, if the hospital has a provider contract with the enrollee's insurer, the hospital can't bill the enrollee except for the normal charges of a copay, coinsurance, or a deductible. And even these charges are barred by some state laws. In essence, the hospital is contractually and legally limited to billing an enrollee as though the insurer had agreed to provide coverage and pay for the care. In fact, a hospital can make an enrollee sign any number of agreements and forms promising to pay for whatever their insurer fails to pay, and it will have no effect on what the hospital can legally bill an enrollee. This includes the form we all sign on entering a hospital or a doctor's office that has us agreeing to pay for whatever our insurance fails to pay. So long as we are an enrollee in a managed-care health insurance plan and the hospital is an in-network provider, the hospital cannot bill us one dollar more than if the insurer had agreed to provide full coverage and pay for the care we receive. The same is true for all other in-network providers.

As strange as all this may sound, it's both the law and the contract reality that all in-network providers (doctors, hospitals, and all the other forms of in-network providers) have voluntarily agreed to accept. Consequently, all an enrollee needs to do when receiving a bill that exceeds these contractual and legal limits is to declare the bill a "legally unenforceable debt." And if a hospital or other in-network provider attempts to enforce such a bill, they can be charged with criminal fraud because they can be readily shown to be fully aware of the restrictions imposed by their provider contract with its Enrollee Hold Harmless clause and the applicable state law.

This is the *"backdoor"* to coverage that the managed-care insurance industry has created, the states have approved, and the in-network providers have agreed to accept. It's also a *"backdoor"* that insurers must keep secret in order to ration the care that you and I can receive.

Justifying a *"Backdoor"* Approach to Care and Coverage:

Because the *"inducement to ration care is the very point"* of managed-care health insurance (Justice David Souter in Pegram), insurers must have some means of overruling the decisions of an enrollee's doctor. And, since the law bars them from doing it directly, they require their in-network doctors, hospitals, and other in-network providers to contractually agree to work for free anytime they render care that the insurer refuses to approve and cover. It's actually quite clever. It's also an excellent way to ensure that a doctor comes around to agreeing with an insurer's view of the most cost-effective (insurance-speak for least costly) approach to care and treatment. However, for this approach to work, the insurer needs time to twist the doctor's arm. And, this is exactly what the insurer's appeal process is designed to do. So why fight to get through the front door when, as an enrollee, you can take your doctor's prescription for care and immediately walk through the insurer's "*backdoor?*" Why waste time appealing a denial of coverage when you can do something that <u>the insurance industry has deliberately designed into your plan</u> and get the very same coverage and cost that you would if you were to win an appeal of coverage? Particularly when winning an appeal is so time consuming and unlikely. Why give your insurer the time it needs to coerce your doctor into accepting the insurer's decision on the care you should or should not be allowed to receive?

Obviously, going through the "*backdoor*" isn't a solution for the nation, because enrollees get the care free of charge, and providers, usually hospitals, have to eat the cost. But, this is the intended design of the insurance industry's provider contracts. Furthermore, in managed-care health insurance, enrollees or their employer actually pay for care in advance. In other words, by going through the "*backdoor*" and demanding the care prescribed by your doctor, you are only following the design of your plan and insisting on the care that has been promised and that you or your employer have already paid for. Our politicians and the insurance industry just don't want you to view it that way. They believe you and all the other enrollees are just too naïve to use the "*backdoor*" that the insurance industry has created, but deliberately hides. In fact, our politicians and the insurance industry are counting on it.

What's more, while provider contracts make it abundantly clear that providers must agree with an insurer's determination of "necessary and appropriate" care in order to get paid, these contracts are equally clear in *requiring* providers to deliver the care that they alone believe is "necessary and appropriate." That's because the only decision insurers are authorized to make on "necessary or appropriate" care is for the distribution of insurance benefits. Furthermore, if these provider contracts actually required physicians and hospitals to accept an insurer's determination of "necessary or appropriate" care, insurers would take on the liability associated with making a medical determination. Something that insurers are highly averse to doing. Therefore, provider contracts don't actually require a doctor or hospital to deliver what an insurer decides is "necessary or appropriate" care. Instead, they require a hospital to provide the care an attending physician (your doctor) prescribes regardless of whether the insurer agrees to pay for it. The doctor and hospital just have to provide their services free of charge, as they have agreed to do by signing the insurer's provider contract.

Stating this as simply as I can, all in-network doctors, hospitals and other in-network providers are legally and contractually required to provide "necessary and appropriate" care in every instance. However, they have to provide it free of charge whenever the insurance company disagrees with what is being prescribed.

Make no mistake, the insurance industry's provider contracts have been meticulously written to allow insurance companies to deny coverage and avoid any liability for their decisions. They effectively force providers to comply with the insurer's *nonmedical* determination of "necessary and appropriate" care while holding the doctor and hospital accountable for *delivering* the medically correct "necessary and appropriate" care. Once again, enrollees are just not supposed to be informed on this small, but very important, point.

So while it's easy to see your doctor, hospital or other provider as innocent victims in this well-constructed scam, you can't afford to do so if you want to be assured of the care you and your family not only need, but are entitled to receice. Your doctor, hospital and any other in-network provider has voluntarily signed these provider contracts and agreed to keep them secret. Yes, the state and the insurance industry have essentially forced them to do so, but they could have said no. They could have done what their profession demands rather than what is financially expedient. And to the credit of some doctors, hospitals and other providers of health care services, they have done exactly that. They have said no to the managed-care scam.

Sandy's doctor provides an excellent example of a doctor following her conscience and professional obligation by refusing to play the managed-care game. Following her inability to properly treat Sandy and numerous other patients, she terminated her provider contracts and went back to school to become a cosmetic surgeon. In so doing, she was able to redefine her practice outside the constraints and contracts of managed care health insurance.

Another example is the nationally renowned Caron Foundation. They reportedly terminated their provider contract with Blue Cross specifically to provide the freedom they needed to treat patients outside the restrictions of the Enrollee Hold Harmless clause. In fact, the head of the foundation's legal department told me that terminating their provider contracts was the only way they could provide care to patients who were being denied coverage. He said Caron had exhausted every other option in trying to find a way around the Enrollee Hold Harmless clause and failed.

The bottom line is that enrollees have to deal with the system as it exists. And because of the mandate in Obamacare, that's now effectively every one of us. So, while going through an insurer's *"backdoor"* for care and coverage may be an imperfect solution for the nation, it's currently the only rational choice for the individual enrollee confronted with an insurer's decision to ration the health care he or she needs. The only other option is to submit to a lengthy and biased appeal process that has been designed to do little more than give an insurer the time it needs to pressure doctors into accepting an insurer's decisions on rationing care. Or per Aetna's Mr. Bertolini, to afford insurers the power to deliver only the care that best supports the *"economy"* and the *"community,"* not the individual enrollee.

The Two Areas of State Law:

Obviously, no two states have exactly the same laws. However, they do have a common structure. Every state has two separate bodies of laws and regulations that affect an enrollee's ability to access health care. One is a state's laws and regulations that oversee the business of insurance and define the requirements for provider contracts. The other is a state's laws and regulations that oversee the delivery of health care services. Where the laws and regulations governing the business of insurance are aimed at protecting the health and stability of the insurance industry, the laws and regulations governing the delivery of health care services are aimed at ensuring the public's access to the highest possible quality of care.

These two different bodies of laws and regulations have very different missions and responsibilities. Because of this, our "*backdoor*" approach to accessing care focuses on the laws and regulations that affect the delivery of health care services rather than the stability of a state's insurance industry. In most states this means using the laws and regulations supported by a department of health rather than those supported by a department of insurance.

While this may seem a trivial point, once again I assure you it is not. For, while a department of health should be willing to enforce its requirements that hospitals provide care whenever it has been properly prescribed and there's an offer to pay for it, a state department of insurance may take a very different position. After all, the insurance department is responsible for both requiring and structuring the provider contracts that allow insurers to ration health care. For this reason it has been my experience that these folks are far more likely to be focused on protecting the authority of an insurance company to ration health care than in overturning an unfair denial of coverage.

Enforcing State Law on Health Services:

Every hospital needs a state license to operate. That license stipulates that hospitals can provide only the care that has been prescribed by a properly licensed physician. The license further stipulates that the hospital must provide properly prescribed care so long as the hospital can provide it and the patient demonstrates a willingness to pay for it.

Please understand that we are not talking about emergency care where hospitals are required to provide care regardless of whether a patient can pay for it. We are talking about situations like Sandy's, where the doctor prescribes care and the hospital refuses to honor the doctor's decision because the insurer is denying coverage. Consequently, once your doctor, or any enrollee's doctor, has prescribed the care that is needed, both state law and the hospital's license require the hospital to provide the care *so long as you, or any other enrollee, demonstrate a willingness to pay for it*. Remember, enrollees have a right to pay. Hospitals just can't take their money. But that's the hospital's problem. You or any other Enrollee are fully within your rights to put your offer to pay in writing and then threaten to both call the state's attorney general and sue that very day if the hospital won't provide the care that is being properly prescribed and required under both state law and the hospital's license. Confrontational, you bet! But a basic tenant in law says that if you don't exercise a right, you lose it.

A great example of what I am describing is when my wife was in the hospital for an irregular heartbeat. I just happened to walk past the nurses' station and overheard a nurse on the phone discussing discharging my wife. This was before I had heard word one from the doctor or had any idea about what was causing my wife's problem. Knowing that a good offense is far better than trying to reverse a decision already made, I leaned over the counter and waited for the nurse to finish her phone call. I then told her that I hoped she would take what I was about to say as nonthreatening as possible. However, she needed to understand that I knew whom she was speaking with and exactly what they were discussing. Furthermore, I said I knew more about what they were discussing than anyone in the hospital or probably the state. *"And if this hospital thinks it's going to discharge my wife before the doctor meets with me and takes direct responsibility for both her care and discharge, the hospital is making the biggest mistake of its life because I will be in my attorney's office before the day is out to file suit. So please don't go there. Don't take us down that road."*

Obviously the poor woman was at a loss for words, but the doctor was in my wife's room within minutes, all smiles and assuring me that *"nothing is going to happen until he and I have met and agreed on the proper course of treatment for my wife."* My response was a simple *"Thank you doctor."*

It's important to remember that confrontation works only when used as a scalpel, not an ax. It needs to be focused and directed at a specific solution. In the case of my wife, all I wanted was a face-to-face meeting with the doctor <u>before any decision was made on discharging her</u>.

A Last Point in Justifying A "Backdoor" Approach to Care & Coverage:

The laws of every state make it crystal clear that: 1.) only a properly licensed doctor can prescribe "necessary and appropriate" health care and 2.) hospitals can only provide properly prescribed "necessary and appropriate" care. Consequently, were your insurer to allow you to pay for care that is available as a "Covered Service" under your plan, but is being denied in a particular instance, the insurer would be providing prima facie evidence that they have deliberately breached the terms of their plan by failing to provide the "necessary and appropriate" care promised by the plan. The only way out of this conundrum would be to have you sign a release prior to allowing you to pay for the care the insurer was refusing to approve. Unfortunately, were the insurer to do that, they would be creating the grounds for charges of extortion and tortious interference with contract for which the insurer would have little if any defense. Furthermore, they would be inviting a judicial review of the Enrollee Hold Harmless clause with all its misrepresentation and its long and broad reach — A review that would all too likely invite a judicial finding that would, almost certainly, limit the insurance industry's power to ration care.

The point is that you, or any other enrollee in a managed-care health plan, are given little or no choice but to access care through the "backdoor" whenever an insurer denies coverage for care that is promised under the terms of their plan. The insurer simply can't afford to let you self-pay for care that they have decided to ration. The risks are far too big. And, their appeal process is intentionally designed to be long, involved and completely misdirected. In short, you can either choose to use the "backdoor" that the insurer has left open, or you can resign yourself or your loved one to the fairness of an appeal process that has been specifically designed to allow your insurer to illegally ration the care you need.

Specific Points to Make the System Work for You:
Cultivate Your Doctor, for He Is the Door to Accessing Care:

Only a properly licensed physician can prescribe health care. So if you can't find a doctor to prescribe the care you need, you will have absolutely no right to receive it, and no hospital or other health care facility will be required to provide it. In fact, state law will actually bar providers from supplying it regardless of your, or anyone else's, willingness to pay for it. Consequently, you need to win your doctor's willing and active support in order to access the care you need and want. In short, *you need to make your doctor your friend and advocate*. And if for some reason this can't be done, you need to find another doctor.

Please remember that it's the doctor-patient relationship that managed-care insurance is intent on destroying. Fortunately, so long as you *vigorously enforce your own doctor-patient relationship*, there is little the system can do to eliminate what is a private and personal relationship in law. After all, it's managed-care that is the enemy, not your doctor.

When Is a Denial of Coverage Most Likely?

While most Americans report that they are satisfied with the care and coverage they receive from their health care plan, there are areas of care where this is not the case. These are areas where you need to anticipate experiencing some form of denial of coverage and rationing. Most notably they are the areas of mental health, drug and alcohol rehabilitation, additional days in hospital, all care that can be labeled cosmetic care, all forms of care that your insurer can label experimental, all care that can be somehow linked to an undisclosed precondition, and all forms of expensive care for the elderly or seriously ill patients. In these areas, you need to anticipate a problem and work with your doctor to avoid it becoming one.

Understand That the Issue Isn't Coverage; It's Whether You "Need" the Care:

While only your doctor can prescribe care, the states have given insurance companies the authority to determine whether the care your doctor is prescribing is "necessary or appropriate" for the purpose of allocating insurance benefits, i.e., rationing health care. Therefore, the game your insurer will be playing when they deny coverage is: 1.) Expecting you to believe that the insurer's physicians are equally authorized to determine the care you should receive, 2.) Believing they can force your doctor to change his or her position over time, and 3.) Knowing that if they can pull you and your doctor into their appeal process, they have won because the issue is cost, not health care.

Unfortunately, doctors almost never put a prescription for care in writing. And even if they do, your insurer knows that: 1.) Your doctor has contractually agreed to "*comply*" with the policies and decisions of the insurer, and 2.) Because the hospital has no hope of getting paid, the doctor will eventually be forced to agree with the insurer.

Most important, always remember that the most significant issue for insurers is inpatient hospitalization and the services that go along with it. That's where the big money resides. Doctors' bills can be an inconvenience. But hospital bills can run into hundreds of thousands of dollars. These are the health care bills that can literally rob you of everything you and your family have, including life itself. It's for this very reason that the book focuses on hospitals far more than the other providers of health care services. However, everything I have said about hospitals applies equally to all the other in-network providers of health care services.

Know the Law Better than Your Hospital/Doctor:

Once your doctor begins to treat you, he or she takes on a duty defined by law and a professional obligation to prescribe and provide the care you need. However, a hospital doesn't have to admit you unless: 1.) Your doctor has admissions rights, 2.) The care is within the hospital's capability, and 3.) There is a reasonable expectation that the hospital can get paid. The first two requirements are both obvious and essentially met automatically. What neither your insurer nor the hospital will ever tell you is that <u>if your insurance company refuses to pay for the care your doctor has prescribed, the hospital is bound by its Provider Contract to provide that care free of charge</u>. The fact that the hospital has signed away its right to bill you in no way lessens your right to pay for the care. You just have to demand your right to pay in order to obligate the hospital, under both contract and law, to provide the care prescribed by your doctor. Consequently, should your insurer refuse to cover the care prescribed by your doctor, you have every right to **immediately**: 1.) Put your offer to pay in writing, 2.) File an immediate complaint with the state's attorney general, and 3.) Threaten to sue the hospital that very day for failing to comply with the laws of the state and the requirements of the hospital's license to operate, knowing full well that if you are ever billed, you are within your rights to refuse the bill as a *"legally unenforceable debt."*

However, do not make the mistake of thinking I am saying that a hospital must provide care free of charge whenever your insurer refuses coverage. The nation's courts have consistently held that hospitals are not in the business of providing free care. So, while it may seem to be no more than a play on words, it is an extremely important point of law to view hospitals as surrendering their right to bill an enrollee rather that being required to provide free care whenever an insurer denies coverage.

Don't Let the System Get Ahead of You (Anticipate and Listen):

Four years ago, our youngest daughter gave birth to two of the prettiest twin girls we could have asked for. However, Kris is quite small, and the twins were both large, healthy babies. As a result, her stomach muscles were badly torn, leaving her with a great deal of pain. Although the solution was simple — it's called a tummy tuck — and can be done only by a cosmetic surgeon, I can't begin to count the number of times the insurer tried to get the term *cosmetic surgery* into the record. Cosmetic surgery is typically an elective procedure not available as a covered service. However, what Kris needed was no more elective surgery than the surgery needed to repair the broken bones in the face of an accident victim. Her insurance company was simply trying to document a means for denying coverage and rationing the care Kris needed.

Anticipating the problem, I took charge of all correspondence and ensured that the record did not include any reference to cosmetic surgery or an elective procedure. That included what her doctor wrote. Not easy, but doable, because, as in most cases, the doctor was a strong advocate for the care Kris needed. The result was that Kris received the coverage and care she was due, and was able to return to full health. Unfortunately, I have to believe that there is no way Kris would have gotten the coverage she deserved if we hadn't anticipated the way her insurer would attempt to deny coverage.

The Threat of Discharge Is Your Constant Enemy:

My wife was recently in the hospital for an irregular heartbeat when I happened to overhear a nurse on the phone discussing her discharge. Now, neither my wife nor I had met with the doctor or had been given any indication of her condition. So I leaned over the nurses' station counter and said the following after she finished her phone call. *"I want what I am going to say to be taken as openly and friendly as possible. However, I know whom you were speaking with and exactly what you were discussing, and I know more about the subject than anyone in this hospital or even in the state. And if this hospital thinks for one moment it's going to discharge my wife before the doctor meets with me and takes direct responsibility for both her care and discharge, the hospital is making the biggest mistake of its life because I will be in my attorney's office to file suit before the day is out. So please don't go there. Don't take us down that road."* I then thanked her for her time and went back to my wife's room. Minutes later the doctor popped into her room all smiles and assurances that nothing would be done until he and I met and agreed on my wife's condition and what needed to be done.

I have repeated this example to make a point. You will never be part of your insurer's determination of "necessary or appropriate" care. That decision will be made by people you will never be allowed to speak to, let alone meet. Your insurer will review your case daily to determine if you should receive one (1) more day of care. Once that decision is "no," the insurer will inform the hospital and your doctor that further coverage is denied, and both the hospital and your doctor will know they won't receive one additional penny for your care and treatment.

The hospital will then explain why you have no choice but to accept termination of care and discharge. Then they get really clever. The hospital will require you to approve your own discharge. Read the fine print of what they require you to sign. For while they will tell you that your doctor has approved the discharge, the doctor is actually only complying with your decision to discharge yourself. The doctor is simply not objecting to your decision.

Of course the hospital will insist that you have no choice but to accept the discharge and that your doctor is in full agreement with the decision. However, watch what happens if you demand to see an order prescribing discharge and signed by your doctor. My experience is that everyone will go silent while the hospital regroups and reconsiders your case.

Consequently, if you only want a day or two of additional time in the hospital rather than an additional lengthy and expensive stay, you can almost certainly get this by simply requiring the hospital to produce an order for discharge signed by your doctor. Doctors are highly averse to signing such an order because they would be accepting personal liability for the decision. This is particularly true for a woman who has given birth and only wants an additional day or two of hospitalization to recuperate.

Or, if you are only looking for an additional day or two of recuperation, you can just tell them you don't feel well enough to leave and refuse to go. What are they going to do? Call the police? And remember, they can't bill you for the extra time. So if you feel you need to stay, stay!

Understand that once your insurer denies additional coverage, the game will be played on their court using their rules. Neither the doctor nor the hospital will be paid from that point on, and the insurer will know that the lack of payment will, in the end, force the doctor and hospital to agree to discharge you or your loved one.

One last, but very important point. It's one thing to obtain some additional recuperative time in a hospital and quite another to force a hospital to continue expensive treatment after your insurer has terminated coverage. Because both the hospital and the doctors will know they can't get paid for further care and treatment, it is my experience that they will be willing to move heaven and earth to limit the cost of any additional care or treatment.

Understand That Transfer to a Nursing Home Means the Loss of Your Doctor:

As a general rule, nursing homes provide only custodial care (essentially room and board). So there is little chance your doctor will have any rights or the ability to attend you or your loved one in a nursing home. That means that even if your doctor wants to retain you as a patient, he or she won't be able to. The doctor won't have the access and support needed to properly attend a patient in a nursing home. Therefore, the only acceptable decision for an attending doctor is to terminate the patient relationship — to stop being your doctor. Anything else would require accepting the liability associated with retaining you as a patient while lacking the access and support needed to attend to your needs. It's something no responsible physician can afford to do.

While I can't prove it, I am absolutely confident that insurance companies count on an enrollee's doctor withdrawing from a case when they force a discharge to a nursing home. The insurer knows the doctor can't follow the patient into the home, and they know the home lacks both a license and the ability to treat a patient. Hence, the insurer can be confident that any appeal of a forced discharge to a nursing home effectively dies at the time of the discharge, as does any request for additional skilled care or treatment. The insurer can simply walk away from the needs and costs of an enrollee. And, in my view, they can be counted on to do exactly that. We experienced it firsthand with Sandy.

Once a patient is discharged to a nursing home they effectively lose access to additional skilled inpatient treatment so long as they remain in the home. They won't have their own doctor and the only doctor the home will have is there solely to deal with emergencies and oversee the general health of the home's residents. In other words, nursing homes provide a perfect dumping ground for insurers seeking to limit their costs. The insurer gets to transfer the full cost of care onto the enrollee and his or her family, and the lack of an *attending physician* means the patient is effectively locked into a no- cost to the insurer status.

Providers Will Close Ranks:

Doctors are generally good people intent on providing all the care a patient needs. Hospitals aren't that much different. Even so, both are hostages to a health care system with an enormous potential for litigation and awards that can run into millions of dollars. For this reason providers can be expected to actively avoid conflict and the liability associated with it. This includes ensuring that the documentation of a patient's needs supports his or her treatment and discharge. Fortunately for doctors and hospitals, and unfortunately for us, this isn't too difficult because most of what a doctor prescribes is done verbally. So while there will always be some documented decisions, it's highly unlikely there will be any smoking guns. When all the smoke clears, one can be pretty certain the records will show the participants (doctors, hospital, and insurer) in full agreement on the appropriate care and treatment a patient should receive. Furthermore, because the appeal process and any form of litigation is long and complex, any opinions or facts that an enrollee might reasonably count on to contest the written record will almost certainly fade away. Simply put, providers *will* close ranks.

Act vs. Wait and Hope:

As I mentioned earlier, there is a familiar saying among attorneys — "No harm, no foul." This is both a common expression and an underlying principle of law. It's particularly true with health care. If you fail to *immediately* press your right to pay for care when unfairly denied coverage, you can expect to lose the opportunity to establish a claim for harm or damage. And without harm or damage, there can be no issue. In other words, if you don't act, you will very likely lose your ability to press your right to access necessary health care.

Threatening to Sue Is Your Greatest Weapon. Having to Sue Is Failure:

While much more could be said here, it's not for this book. After ten years in court, I am more than convinced that suing is the last thing you want to do. However, the last thing your insurance company wants is to have the Enrollee Hold Harmless clause and the many issues it creates called into question. They certainly won't want our "*back door*" approach to coverage debated in open court. But if you do sue for the right to pay, as we did, you can be assured they will fight you tooth and nail because you will be attacking the entire industry and the very foundation of managed-care's ability to ration health care.

My strong suggestion and the actual purpose of this book is to arm individual enrollees with the information they need to circumvent the system and leave the suing to the class action attorneys and advocate groups with the skill, power and money needed to hold the industry accountable.

Some Definitions You Will Need:

If you are anything like me, you will be tempted to skip this section as just a list of boring definitions. However, I implore you not to do it here. The fraud I have described in this book is so grounded in the industry's use of misleading terms and procedures that there is simply no way to understand the care and coverage you are owed from a managed-care health plan without committing these definitions to memory.

Appeal Process:

An insurer's process for appealing a denial of coverage is one that is intentionally lengthy, wrongly directed and largely designed to give the insurer the time and cover it needs to enforce its decisions on rationing health care. By wrongly directed I mean that an appeal should focus on the owner of a plan and not the enrollee who is typically simply accessing the plan of his or her employer. Also, unless you file a timely formal appeal of a denial of coverage or immediately pursue coverage through your plan's "*backdoor*," you will lose the right to do either.

Benefit:

The specific care that is defined as available in an *employer's health plan* but secretly contingent on whether the insurer agrees to pay for it in any particular instance.

Benefit Package:

The entire inventory of benefits that are provided for an employee by an employer, health insurance being but one component of what is typically a multi-element package of benefits.

Benefit Period:

The period of time that is covered contractually by an employer's plan, which is typically one calendar year beginning on January 1 and ending on December 31 of that same year.

Coinsurance Amount:

An enrollee's portion of what an insurer is expected to pay for a covered service, typically a percentage of the insurer's cost, which is set within a managed-care health plan. Note that insurance companies and state law may allow a coinsurance payment to be collected at the time of service. However, as explained earlier in this book, there is no way a provider can determine the correct amount of coinsurance until after an insurer has reviewed the provider's bill. And there is no way you can determine the correct *coinsurance* until you have been provided the details of the insurer's provider contract along with a copy of the insurer's determination of coverage for each individual charge that make up a provider's bill.

Copayment Amount:

A specific dollar amount that an enrollee pays directly to a provider at the time care is provided. Copayments are typically a small charge and established by the specific plan an enrollee is entitled to use. They are most often associated with doctor visits or pharmaceutical coverage. As a general rule, copayments do not count toward an enrollee's deductible or coinsurance.

Coverage:

This is a term for which insurers have two (2) **very different definitions**:

> 1) All of the "necessary and appropriate" health care that is ***available*** under a plan when an insurer promotes the total "*coverage*" of their plan.
>
> *and*
>
> 2) The limits to coverage in a specific "*instance*" when the insurer rations care by overruling the attending physician and "*denying coverage*" for the very care that is ***available*** under an enrollee's plan.

Covered Services:

All the "necessary and appropriate" health care that an enrollee needs or receives. Please note that even if an insurer denies coverage for care that an attending physician has determined to be "necessary and appropriate," the care ***remains a "Covered Service"*** under the terms of the insurer's plan, the insurer's provider contract, and state law. The insurer is simply enforcing its state sanctioned authority to ration health care by denying what it has promised as a "*Covered Service*," in a particular instance.

So long as the care your doctor is prescribing isn't an electable cosmetic procedure or an experimental treatment, it's a "*Covered Service*," regardless of whether your insurer agrees to cover and pay for it. This is an extremely important point because any attempt to deny coverage will be cloaked in an insurer's assertion that the care your doctor is prescribing is outside the coverage of your plan. They will want you to believe that they are simply acting on the limits of your plan rather than refusing to accept the medical decisions of your doctor.

Remember, they have promised all the "necessary and appropriate" health care and coverage you need. They have even structured their provider contracts to ensure you get that level of care and coverage. However, by misrepresenting the definition of "*Covered Services*" and hiding the details of their provider contracts, they keep you and all other enrollees in the dark, adrift in a rigged appeal process and subject to their scheme to muzzle your doctor and ration the health care they have promised. As Aetna's Mr. Bertolini so aptly put it, your health care needs must "*capitulate*" to the needs that the insurer believes are more important.

Deductible Payment:

A specific dollar amount established by a managed-care plan that must be paid by the enrollee prior to the insurer paying for a "*Covered Service*." Once again, there is absolutely no way for you to determine an appropriate amount of a "Deductible Payment" until you have been provided the details of the insurer's provider contract and the insurer's review of the provider's list of individual charges.

Denial of Coverage:

Contrary to what insurers would like you to believe, this is not a denial of "*Coverage*." It's a refusal to pay for a "*Covered Service*." The insurer simply decides that you don't need the care or that it's too expensive and refuses to pay for it, i.e., rations the care your doctor believes you need.

Emergency Care:

We all have a right to emergency health care at a hospital, regardless of our ability to pay. At least so long we seek emergency care from a hospital that has agreed to work within the Federal Government's Medicare system. But that is about as much as most of us know about our right to emergency care. That's largely because insurers and participating hospitals discourage the use of this type of care. The insurer doesn't want us to use it because it strips away their ability to ration care through their *"Precertification"* process. And hospitals don't want us to use it because it creates a drain on their finances. As a result, both organizations work to minimize the care an emergency patient can receive as well as the time they can remain in an ER (a hospital emergency room). In essence, both organizations see themselves having to limit the care that an enrollee can receive in an ER. Or stated more simply, they have a need to limit the cost of emergency care. And, that would be understandable if they didn't use managed-care's misrepresentation and fraud to pursue that need.

I'm certain I could write an entire book on the misrepresentation and fraud in emergency care. I could certainly write a long and dedicated chapter. But that would be outside the focus of this book. Instead, let me simply provide the elements of emergency care that an enrollee needs to understand to make the most of a very misrepresented and misunderstood system.

1.) Emergency care is merely what its name states — the care needed to address and *stabilize* an emergency condition. It is not meant or designed to provide in-depth care or curative treatment. More specifically, *"emergency service is any health care service provided to evaluate and/or treat any medical condition such that a prudent layperson possessing an average knowledge of medicine and health, believes that immediate unscheduled medical care is required"*(American College of Emergency Physicians).

2.) The common belief that anyone needing *health care* can receive it in a hospital ER is absolutely false. In fact it's not even close, even if you have a managed-care insurance plan that promises full coverage.

3.) While you can't be refused emergency care, the only requirement of an ER is that they conduct an appropriate medical examination and then *stabilize* your condition or transfer you to another medical facility with the capability to address the emergency.

4.) While the definition of *stabilize* has proven highly controversial, there is little question that it does not include any preventive care or any curative treatment. It simply requires an ER to address what is an *imminent* threat to an individual's health. *To provide such medical treatment . . . as may be necessary to assure, within reasonable medical probability, that no material deterioration of the condition is likely to result*, (American Medical Association).

5.) An ER will almost certainly try to convince you that they are separate from the hospital and limited to the staff on duty in the ER. Neither is true. The law governing emergency care applies to hospitals, not their ER. Therefore, all the staff and capabilities of the hospital are available to treat a patient's emergency condition.

6.) The most critical part of receiving appropriate care in an ER is the classification of the emergency. Do not allow this determination to be made without your participation. Furthermore, <u>insist that the examining doctor sign the determination of your emergency condition</u>.

7.) Understand that a hospital receives a single dollar

amount for your emergency, regardless of whether you are in and out of the ER in an hour or remain there for days. Consequently, the staff will be doing all they can to limit the care you receive and your time in the ER. The only way this will change is to be formally admitted to the hospital.

8.) If you have any concern about being prematurely discharged or undertreated, insist that the attending physician take personal responsibility for the discharge by <u>signing an *order* for the discharge</u>.

The bottom line is that while the people who work in emergency rooms are good people, the system that they are forced to work under is anything but open and honest. So, if you are in need of care and an ER appears to be ignoring that need or has you headed for a premature discharge, you are going to have to be both knowledgeable and demanding to get the care you need.

Enrollee Hold Harmless Clause:

Specific language that all the states mandate for inclusion in the provider contracts that insurers are required to have with each of their in-network providers. The following three points are meant to summarize the effect that these contracts have on the individual enrollee, i.e., you. However the list is in no way intended to be complete. Unfortunately, the only way to obtain that complete list is to be given access to the specific provider contract an insurer is enforcing.

In general, all Enrollee Hold Harmless clauses;

1.) Bar providers from billing an enrollee for covered services except in a few specifically stated instances,

194

2.) Bar providers from contracting privately with enrollees for any necessary care an insurer has refused to approve and cover.
3.) Provide the primary enforcement mechanism for denying coverage and rationing health care.
4.) *"Sever"* an enrollee's doctor-patient relationship.

Medical Records:

Contrary to what you may have been led to believe, you not only have a right to see your medical records, but to also receive a copy under the federal HIPAA law. Furthermore, providers can't charge more than the actual reproduction cost. In Pennsylvania, state law sets a maximum charge for copying medical records of $1.42 per page for the first 20 pages, $1.05 for the next 40 pages, and 34 cents for anything beyond that. In New York, state law limits providers from charging more than 75 cents per page, even when the actual expense exceeds that amount.

Necessary or Appropriate Care:

A term the insurance industry wants us to believe has only one definition. Unfortunately, managed-care health insurance companies, once again, use two very different definitions:

1.) An insurer's *financial determination* of the care an enrollee should receive in order to ration care.

2.) An attending physician's *medical determination* of the care an enrollee needs to receive *as a matter of law*.

In fact, it's the use of these two separate definitions that lies at the core of managed-care's power to ration health care and their outstanding financial success

Non-Covered Services:

The services that are <u>specifically</u> excluded from the "Covered Services" of a managed-care plan, i.e., the services that are not *"available"* from a plan under any circumstances. These "Non-Covered Services" are typically limited to elective cosmetic procedures and experimental treatments.

Precertification:

An insurer's process for reviewing all but emergency care prior to the actual rendering of care. Although the insurance industry would love to have us stop here, the term *"Precertification"* speaks volumes in terms of proving that the insurance industry is involved in a deliberate fraud aimed at circumventing the law. Remember, only a properly licensed attending physician can certify the care a patient needs, i.e., your doctor. And once that properly licensed physician certifies the care that is needed, a hospital must provide it because an enrollee, on entering the hospital, signs a form promising to pay for any care the insurer fails to cover. It's the law in every state in the country. The only exception is for care that is outside the hospital's capability. But even then the hospital is obligated to transfer the enrollee to another hospital that can provide care that has been properly prescribed and the patient has agreed to pay for. However, if the insurer can intervene before the doctor *"certifies"* the care that is needed, it can inform the doctor and the hospital that they won't get paid if they provide that level of care, i.e., the level of care the insurer claims the doctor is *only considering.* And since a doctor isn't likely to force a hospital to provide free care, even if the doctor is willing to go unpaid, the insurer can be confident that the doctor will, in time, accept the insurer's decision on the level of care that should or should not be provided. Simply put, precertification isn't a determination of coverage as your insurer would have you believe. It's the insurer's process for strong-arming your doctor into agreeing with the insurer's determination of the care you should or should not be *allowed* to receive, i.e., the rationing of the care you need and have every right to access under the law.

By labeling the process "Precertification," the insurer asserts that anything your doctor prescribes prior to the insurers "Precertification" constitutes no more than preliminary thoughts leading to the doctor's actual *certification* of "necessary and appropriate" care.

Provider Contract:

A state-mandated contract between a managed-care insurance company and each of its in-network providers that:

1.) Severs the enrollee's doctor-patient relationship.
2.) Defines the *actual* access that enrollees will have to "necessary and appropriate" health care.
3.) Limits what the providers can bill.
4.) Establishes discounted pricing for the insurer.
    5.) Is filed away and labeled a secret document so that enrollees will never see any part of its controlling terms, conditions, and pricing. **See Appendix 8 for a representative example.**

Rescissions:

A long standing insurance industry practice of terminating an enrollee's participation in a plan for what the insurer claims is a failure to disclose pertinent health care information or a precondition. It has been described by whistle blowers like Wendell Potter as the means the industry uses to keep their plans free of the most seriously ill and costly patients. Something Obamacare should end.

Uninsured:

Individuals without insurance but with *unrestricted access* to all "necessary and appropriate" health care. This is an absolutely huge point. Because, so long as you are uninsured, you have an absolute right to access all the care your doctor believes you need and you are willing to pay for. However, the moment your employer awards you a benefit package with a managed-care health plan, all that constitutionally protected right to access health care vanishes — along with a right to a private and personal doctor-patient relationship with *your* very own doctor.

Utilization Review:

A process by which the insurer has the authority to review the status of every enrollee receiving care and decide whether to continue that level of care and coverage. In fact, an insurance company's authority to conduct these reviews is so absolute that both the review and findings can be applied retroactively. In other words, an insurer can conduct its review at any time and decide that any ongoing care, or even care that was earlier "Precertified" and rendered, does not qualify as "necessary and appropriate" and therefore does not qualify for the insurer's coverage and payment. The insurer can even force a provider to return money that it received for care that was "Precertified" and rendered months in the past. What's more, in all these retroactive denials of coverage, the insurer's provider contracts state that the provider (hospital or doctor) *"shall not bill or charge Insurer or Enrollee."* See Utilization Review, Section 5, Appendix 8. More specifically, see provisions 5.8, 5.9, and 5.10. Please note that these restrictions on billing enrollees are in addition to the restrictions imposed by the Enrollee Hold Harmless clause.

By having doctors and hospitals sign provider contracts, the insurer grants itself the power to deny payment any time it decides there has been a mistake, it has to reduce costs, or it is failing to meet the financial objectives of its investors.

I could stop here, but a while back I heard Dr. Sonjay Gupta on public radio describe an excellent example of a utilization review and how insurers and providers twist the definitions of key terms to serve their own interests.

Dr. Gupta interviewed a woman who had undergone extensive throat surgery to relieve a condition that was restricting her ability to breathe. She explained that her insurance company had "Precertified" the procedure and then months later (I believe it was nine months after the operation) informed her that they were denying coverage and refusing to pay for the operation. The hospital then billed her for more than a million dollars.

Dr. Gupta's question was, *"How is this possible?"* The woman had simply gotten the care her insurer had agreed to cover. Dr. Gupta said he was completely mystified and promised to devote future programming to the issue. Unfortunately, the answer to Dr. Gupta's question, while readily available, is probably one he will never share with his radio audience. In fact I wrote to him with the answer to his question and haven't heard a word from him. Not that this surprises me.

To answer Dr. Gupta's question of *"How is this possible,"* one needs only read the terms and conditions of the provider contract that the hospital signed with the woman's insurance company. Of course, as I have said repeatedly, no one is going to willingly make that provider contract available. However, rest assured it contains provisions that, for all practical purposes, mirror provisions 5.8, 5.9, and 5.10 in Appendix 8. In fact, insurers typically publish a manual on how these utilization reviews are conducted. Once again, however, these manuals are only available to a select few within the health care community. All that said, the bottom line is that managed-care insurance companies (and almost certainly the insurer of Dr. Gupta's guest) use their provider contracts to give themselves unlimited power to deny payment to a doctor or hospital whenever the insurer chooses to find a specific course of treatment or care not "necessary and appropriate."

The only issue open for discussion is whether the hospital had a right to bill Dr. Gupta's guest once coverage was withdrawn and the insurer had taken back what it had paid for the woman's operation. The answer is an unequivocal "No." However, in the case of Dr. Gupta's quest we are talking about a loss of over a million dollars — a sum the hospital could be expected to do everything possible to recover.

Fortunately for both the insurer and the hospital, there was a simple solution, albeit a deliberately fraudulent one. The hospital only had to claim that the insurer's denial of coverage made the operation a *"Noncovered Service."* After all, who would think it could be anything else?

By allowing everyone to conclude that the woman's operation had become a N*oncovered Service,"* the insurer freed the hospital to bill the woman and pursue payment through the courts. Even better for the insurer, this guaranteed that the matter would center on whether they had a right to deny coverage based on their "contractual" determination of "necessary and appropriate" health care. This was a clear win for the insurer because their provider contract provides this very authority. It's also a clear win for the hospital because who would think that the patient isn't responsible for what her insurer fails to pay?

Unfortunately for Dr. Gupta and his guest, the answer to the woman's problem is one neither of them is likely to see or hear outside of this book. Regardless of what the hospital and the woman's insurer would like her to believe, the operation she received remained a "Covered Service" by law and contract, in spite of the insurer's utilization review and its decision to retroactively deny coverage. Therefore, the hospital had no right to bill the woman. The Enrollee Hold Harmless clause, as well as numerous other provisions in the hospital's provider contract, make this point crystal clear. Dr. Gupta's guest could have simply declared the hospital's bill a *legally unenforceable debt* and sent it back unpaid. At a bare minimum, she, or her attorney, should have demanded the hospital produce a copy of their provider contract to prove they had the right to bill her. Imagine the mess that would have created for the hospital. Their provider contract not only bars any such billing but also prohibits the hospital from disclosing the details of the contract.

And so we come, once again, to the purpose of this book. There is just no way Dr. Gupta's guest could have been expected find knowledgeable help in protecting her from the hospital's attorneys. These were folks pursuing a million dollars. Additionally, they were undoubtable smart people who had executed this type of deception many times. Therefore, it's reasonable to assume that they were not only experts at this type collection, but brash and intimidating. Even worse, these attorneys had the power of what everyone would view as common sense to support their arguments.

Unfortunately, I have yet to find a private attorney with enough understanding of the system to provide the help the woman needed or a factual explanation to Dr. Gupta. I can say this with great confidence because I was immersed in just such a battle for ten years and never found an attorney who understood the issue. Hopefully, this book will provide what I couldn't find and Dr. Gupta's guest needed so desperately. If my memory serves me right, she eventually settled with the hospital for something like $300,000 when she could have easily proven the bill was a *legally unenforceable debt* and charged the hospital with criminal fraud if it continued to pursue her for any part of the $1,000,000 bill.

FOURTEEN

···......................................

"The law does not pretend to punish everything that is dishonest. That would seriously interfere with business:"
Clarence Darrow

The Decision We Face as a Nation

Under the guise of controlling the rising cost of health care, the managed-care insurance industry and our new mega-hospitals are waging a calculated and deliberate war to eliminate the doctor-patient relationship as we have known it. In fact, only today I heard a radio advertisement for Wellspan Health — a health care holding corporation that virtually controls health care services in south central Pennsylvania and seventeen similar locations across the country. Their radio ad and webpage herald that "*We are introducing a whole new doctor-patient relationship through a team of doctors*" and "*working to create healthier populations*" and "*working with physicians to improve the community health*," (Wellspan's July 3, 2014 radio ad and their Wellspan.org website). Now *please* remember the words of Aetna CEO Mark Bertolini where he states the our <u>individual</u> rights must "**_capitulate_** *to the needs of the community*" and the health care system must be redesigned to focus on "*population health management*" and to "*improve the health of the population in a way that provides a more valuable input into the* *economy of the country.*"

How can the choice we face be clearer? For, nowhere in the Wellspan's ad or in Aetna's ever-so-clear plans for the nation's future do they bother to mention the rights and needs of the individual — the rights and needs of you and me and the elderly couple across the street. The rights that each and every one of us have to our very own private and personal doctor-patient relationship and the freedom to access the health care we choose regardless of what Aetna, our mega-hospitals or politicians believe is best for business and the economy — the very rights that our men in uniform have died to protect for more than 250 years. However, to be fair to the insurance industry, the decision to initiate this war has been forced on them, and it's one they can only wage in secret.

When Congress passed the 1973 HMO Act, they assigned the managed-care insurance industry, the task of reining in the unacceptable rise in the national cost of health care. And, while one might argue that no one saw this leading to the systematic and surreptitious rationing that we have today, it doesn't change the fact that this is where we find ourselves.

Because the rise in the cost of health care has been driven by an explosion in medical technology and the aspirations of citizens for a longer and better life, insurers can no longer control costs by simply negotiating greater and greater discounts from in-network providers. Furthermore, these in-network providers are more and more becoming mega-hospital organizations that demand greater and greater revenue and profits. As Lynn Jennings, CEO of WeCare TLC so aptly put it, "*When an employer sits down with his health care providers — the broker, the insurer, the physician, the hospital, the drug and device firms — everyone in the room wants it to cost more — and they're all positioned to make it happen.*" Consequently, insurers, and Congress have found themselves needing something else to control the rising cost of health care. Unfortunately, that something else can only be rationing. And, rationing for managed-care health insurance absolutely demands an ability to overrule attending physicians for determining "necessary and appropriate" health care.

The bottom line is that the managed-care insurance industry — HMO, PPO, POS, or whatever acronym is used — has to ration health care. And to do that, they have to sever the doctor-patient relationship so that *they* can determine the care that is needed rather than the attending physician (your doctor). In other words, the insurer becomes the prescriber of care, and the physician becomes simply a highly trained technician charged with delivering the care an insurer has prescribed. As Aetna's CEO, Mr. Bertolini, so aptly put it, "___It really requires the providers to trust us in ways that they've never had to trust us___."

If there remains any doubt that this is where our health care system is headed, one doesn't have to look very far for proof. The news is full of articles reporting the fierce competition between insurers and mega-hospitals to become one-stop shops that dominates health care delivery in a particular area. A one-stop shop that makes private physicians (our doctors) their employees — employees who owe their allegiance and careers to their employer and not you or me or any individual patient.

That's the health care industry's strategy for redefining the doctor-patient relationship. By bringing doctors together as a team under their employer, the enrollee no longer has a doctor who can be held responsible for the care he or she receives. That long held responsibility is now spread over a team that can't be held responsible for delivering anything more than the most cost effective average standard of care as a matter of law. And it is very well held that their employer (insurance company or mega-hospital) can't be held for rendering anything more either. They are both completely free to ration the care you and I receive. As a result, the care that you and I are allowed to receive becomes the least expensive average standard of care based on the needs of the "*community*" and the "*economy*." As Aetna CEO Mark Bertolini argued in his interview with Dylan Scott, "*I think everyone does realize that it's time to change.*"

This is the core of the choice we face as a nation. It isn't a question of whether we need some form of rationing. We already have it. Anyone familiar with the projected cost of health care will readily understand why we have it. However, just because we need some form of rationing to control the national cost of health care doesn't mean we need to surrender our doctor-patient relationship. In fact, surrendering our doctor-patient relationship as a way to cut the national cost of health care makes no more sense than surrendering the attorney-client relationship as a way to cut the national cost of frivolous lawsuits.

In order to protect their authority to regulate health insurance, the states have adopted the recommendations of the NAIC (the National Association of Insurance Commissioners). These recommendations require insurers to have a provider contract with every in-network provider of health care services. Furthermore, the contracts must contain an Enrollee Hold Harmless clause. And while these contracts along with their Enrollee Hold Harmless clause have provided the protection the states wanted to regulate insurance, they have also made the managed-care insurance industry and the states partners in severing the doctor-patient relationship without notice, process, or any form of consent by the individual enrollee. In essence, it can be readily shown that the states and the insurance industry have cooperated for the sole purpose of denying enrollees their constitutional right to contract, process, liberty, and privacy in their doctor-patient relationship and in *accessing* health care at their own expense. All for the purpose of rationing the health care services an individual enrollee can receive.

It's this conflict between the heath care industry's need to ration health care and the limits our laws place on interfering in a private and personal doctor-patient relationship that forms the crux of the problem facing the nation and the managed-care insurance industry. Because insurers have to both ration care and do it secretly, they and their in-network providers must operate outside the law, particularly federal law. And, because Obamacare now directly exposes the entire managed-care operation to federal law, we are faced with a huge dilemma. Something has to change. Either we change the laws that guarantee the sanctity of the doctor-patient relationship and our constitutional right to access health care at our own expense or we force the managed-care insurance industry to change how they ration health care <u>while respecting the sanctity of the doctor-patient relationship</u>. It's just that simple.

Because Obamacare mandates that everyone have acceptable managed-care health insurance, the entire business of managed-care insurance is, for the first time, directly exposed to the full range of federal law. Furthermore, the right to a personal and private doctor-patient relationship in *accessing and contracting for* necessary health care is grounded in the explicit language of the U. S. Constitution. Consequently, the current practice of rationing health care by secretly interfering in an enrollee's doctor-patient relationship cannot survive. The contrast between what the law allows and the industry's scheme for rationing is simply too great. After all, *"The key ingredient in learning the truth is to ask the right questions,"* U. S. Senator Daniel Pactric Moynihan. In essence, the only question is when and how change will occur.

Fortunately, for those unable or unwilling to wait for this change to occur, there is a gaping hole in the current managed-care system that allows enrollees to circumvent the severing of their doctor-patient relationship. I call it the *"backdoor"* to care and coverage. Unfortunately, it's a wide open *backdoor* only if an enrollee knows how to use it.

Enrollees need only demand to pay for any care that is being unfairly denied for coverage, sign anything the provider requires to guarantee payment, and then declare the bill a "legally unenforceable debt" once he or she has received the care they are due under the law. It's in accord with the laws in every state in the country. You just have to demand your right to pay, knowing they can't bill you, and hold the hospital accountable under the law and the terms of their provider contract for delivering the care *your* doctor has prescribed.

For those who remain convinced that reform of our health care system cannot involve any form of rationing, you really need to pull your head out of the sand. Establishing a health care system that allows everyone to receive all the care they believe they need makes no more sense than reforming Social Security to allow everyone to receive all the income they believe they need. In both cases the cost would be uncontrollable and beyond anything the nation can afford. Consequently, *the issue isn't whether to have rationing. It's how to have rationing that provides an affordable baseline for reasonable care and coverage and also: 1.) Retains our constitutional right to our very own private and personal doctor-patient relationship and 2.) Preserves our individual right to access more care than private or government insurance can or should provide.*

A Last Word:

While I can't prove it, it makes all the sense in the world that a primary reason behind the insurance industry's support for Obamacare was the recognition that they would codifying the Enrollee Hold Harmless clause in federal law. In other words, they would be embodying the Clause and their power to ration health care so deeply into the laws and policies of the nation that there would be no way of going back. Dare I say it? Aetna's Mr. Mark Bertolini's "*standing wave phenomenon.*" A force so powerful that once organized and launched on the American people, the nation's acceptance of the insurance industry's power to openly ration health care would be a fait accompli.

FIFTEEN

....

"Where you stand depends on where you sit:"

Miles Law

The Decision You & I Face

While passage of Obamacare may have broadened the nation's access to health insurance, it has most certainly increased the power of the insurance industry to rob you and me of our doctor, ration critically needed care and steal us blind with fraudulent bills. This isn't an author's opinion. It isn't even a forecast of a likely outcome. It's the hard reality of a system that the insurance industry and our government have been secretly building for more than thirty years — a system that sacrifices the rights of the individual for the insurance industry's profitability and government's need to reduce the cost of health care.

Consider what we can say with certainty about where health care is headed in the United States. We know that: 1.) We have to reduce the national cost of health care, 2.) We have to significantly increase the number of people who can receive care, and 3.) The country's population is exploding with seniors who will need the most expensive care of their lives and the poor who can't afford to pay for either care or insurance. However, we are told not to worry because the solution to successfully meeting these challenges lies in simply making the system more *"efficient."* In fact, the news is full of these assurances, i.e., the numerous reports on how insurance companies, our new mega-hospitals, physicians and government are all focused on improving the *"efficiency"* in health care. However, what we don't hear is exactly what improving *"efficiency"* means. And, we certainly don't hear what it means for the average individual, i.e., the you and me and our loved-ones. We are not even provided with a definition for the term. Instead, much like the promises of your plan, your doctor and the best care that modern science has to offer, we are left to assume that improving *"efficiency"* is a good thing for both the nation and the individual needing health care.

Unfortunately, this is just another example of where we are being deliberately misled. *"We have no definition of true efficiency,"* conclusion of the national conference "Efficiency in Health Care" May 23-24, 2006. *"To date no broad consensus has emerged on how to define efficiency for the health care system,"* Pay for Performance in Health Care, RTI Press, March 2011. *"Efficiency in health care: does anyone really know what they mean,"* James F. Burgess, Jr., Department of Health Policy and Management, School of Public Health, Boston University, April 2012. And, *"We have no definition for true efficiency,"* Looking for Healthcare Efficiency in all the Wrong Places, blog.teletracting.com, June 2014.

This is not to imply that there aren't unnecessary costs in the nation's health care system. There clearly are. However, if there isn't a clear definition of *"efficiency"* then exactly what are all the participants in our health care system pursuing so aggressively?

They are pursuing lower production costs as any for-profit enterprise must do to drive profits in a capitalistic system. However, here they are doing it in a market where growth must be artificially constrained by government while the need for health care services is expanding at an unprecedented rate. The undeniable result is that the participants in our health care system are pursuing ever greater rationing of what you and I can receive in the way of "necessary and appropriate" health care. And, they are doing it under the guise of improving *"efficiency."* In fact, it's not even a choice. They are being forced to ration the care we can receive.

For those who doubt what I am saying, please go to the internet and Google health care rationing in the United States. The list of references will be endless. And, all arguing that: 1.) rationing already exists in the Unites States, 2.) rationing is absolutely essential in order to control the cost of care, and 3.) it has to be carefully hidden from the American people. Then, Google all statements denying the rationing of health care in the United States. You won't find a single suitable reference. I certainly didn't.

The bottom line here is that where health care is concerned, there can be no limits to health care and coverage under the managed care industry's promise of all the "necessary and appropriate" care an individual needs and our individual Constitutional right to access all the care we can pay for.

The problem is obvious. While we have inherent spending limitations that require rationing, we also have a culture, guaranteed legal rights and a managed care insurance system where there can be no limits on the care we receive. Therefore, there can be no rationing. In fact, our culture, legal rights, and insurance system don't even allow room for a discussion of rationing except to condemn it in the worst of terms.

It's these two basic imperatives that are shaping our health care system and its pursuit of ever greater *"efficiency"* — the unavoidable need to ration health care and our American culture, law and insurance system of no limits. Given our deep-seated need to simultaneously cling to both of these clearly incompatible imperatives, our only option is to pursue unavoidable rationing in a way that allows us to deny that rationing is even occurring. Simply stated, to ration care in a way that allows the health care industry and government to declare that there are no limits on the care we can receive. In essence, to ration secretly, i.e., to improve the "efficiency" of how health care is delivered.

This is the reality of what we face as individuals. In fact it's proof of the old adage that *"where you stand depends on where you sit."* While our politicians and the heads of our health care institutions may very well believe they are exercising the only option open to the nation, that does not mean that they are acting in the best interests of the individual needing health care. They clearly are not and that is the nexus of the decision that faces each of us in accessing the care that we and are families will need. We can either accept the system with its ever greater "efficiency" and put our trust in politicians and the insurance industry, or we can choose to walk a different road. We can choose to demand the access to health care that is guaranteed us in both law and contract. We can pursue care as individuals and outside the rationing that has been so carefully hidden within the U. S. health care system.

I have already made my decision. After ten years of litigating the issue and failing to get any help what-so-ever from the courts, my state, or Washington (see Appendixes 5,6,7,12 & 13), the decision was easy. I had learned that by applying the information in this book on how our health care system actually works, I can protect myself and my family regardless of the system's efforts at *"efficiency"* and rationing. In fact, there is no question in my mind that I can guarantee us the highest level of care and coverage our system has to offer. The question then become, can you?

Fortunately, the real power of this book rests not with what you and the American people can look to from Congress or even the courts. It rests with the power that the individual enrollee can exert on the system by simply demanding his or her rights. To, at a minimum, insist on a single responsible doctor of your own choosing in a true doctor-patient relationship, obtain care and coverage through the *"backdoor"* whenever it's being unfairly denied, have hospitals take direct responsibility for their actions by insisting that a doctor sign an order that supports the hospital's decisions on the care you receive, and demand a bill that complies with the Enrollee Hold Harmless clause and all the other applicable contract and legal restrictions on billing an enrollee. That's the real power of this book. It's what one small voice can do for reform that all the advocates, Congress, our politicians, the heads of industry and the legal community have either failed to do or refused to do for more than twenty years! Or as simply as I can state it, the book not only provides the means for you to obtain the care and coverage you and your family are due, but it makes the individual enrollee in managed care health insurance (you) a primary voice in the push for true reform. Furthermore, it makes our collective individual voices proof positive that the system is just Too Big to Be Legal!

Finally, I need to again remind readers that I am not an attorney, nor am I representing myself as an expert on the laws that affect the delivery of health care and insurance in the United States. This book is solely the author's attempt to share what ten years of litigation and the death of Sandra Lobb have taught him about managed-care health insurance. Therefore, everything I have written should be reviewed by a competent attorney before putting the contents of the book into practice.

Appendix

Appendix #1

Pennsylvania's Enrollee Hold Harmless Clause

Hospital/Doctor agrees that in no event, including but not limited to non-payment by Insurance Company, Insurance Company's insolvency or breach of this agreement, shall Hospital, one of its subcontractors, or any of its employees or independent contractors bill, charge, collect a deposit from, seek compensation, remuneration or reimbursement from, or have any recourse against a Subscriber or persons other than the insurance company acting on behalf of Subscriber for Covered Services provided pursuant to this Agreement. This provision shall not prohibit the collection of coinsurance, co-payments or charges for Non-Covered Services. Hospital/Doctor further agrees that (1) this provision shall survive the termination of this Agreement regardless of the cause giving rise to termination and shall be construed to be for the benefit of the Subscribers, and that (2) this provision supersedes any oral or written contrary agreement now existing or hereafter entered into between Hospital/Doctor and Subscribers or persons acting on their behalf. Hospital/Doctor may not change, amend or waive this provision without prior written consent of the Insurance Company. Any attempt to change, amend or waive this provision are void.

Appendix #2

NAIC's Suggested Enrollee Hold Harmless Language

The requirement of Subsection B shall be met by including a provision substantially similar to the following:

Provider agrees that in event, including but not limited to, nonpaymeny by health maintenance organization or intermediary organization, insolvency of the health maintenance organization or intermediary organization, or breach of this agreement shall the provider bill, charge, collect a deposit from, seek compensation, remuneration or reimbursement from, or have any recourse against a covered person or a person (other than the health maintenance organization or intermediary organization) acting on behalf of the covered person for covered services provided pursuant to this agreement. This agreement does not prohibit the provider from collecting coinsurance, deductibles, copayments or services in excess of limits as specifically provided in the evidence of coverage, or fees for uncovered services delivered on a fee-for-service basis to covered persons.

Any bill sent to a covered person shall include the following:

Notice: You are not responsible for any amount owed by your insurer.

Appendix #3

Author's Letter to Edwin J. Feulner

Frank H Lobb
P. O. Box 242
Nottingham, PA 19362

Dr. Edwin J. Feulner, Pres.
The Heritage Foundation
214 Massachusetts Ave., NE
Washington, DC 20002

May 1, 2012

Dear Dr. Feulner:

The health care insurance industry and state regulatory agencies have long hidden the fact that when an employer gives an employee managed care health insurance (as essentially all employers do) they secretly surrender the employee's right to purchase any necessary care the insurer, for whatever reason, refuses to approve. And they do it so well that it took me ten (10) years of intense litigation to dig out the details and the necessary proof. The bottom line is that the material I obtained dramatically changes managed care health insurance and the law surrounding it. Even more interesting, when I came to the Heritage Foundation for help in this effort, your Dr. Moffit dropped me like a hot rock as soon as he had the details of where I was headed, i.e., proof that each of us have the right to purchase the care prescribed by our doctor that can't be secretly set aside by the state or an insurance company. Interestingly, the Canadian hero Dr. Jacques Chaoulli, had the same experience I did when he sought help from Dr. Moffit and Heritage. --- And yes, I am a registered Republican!

To insure you don't see me as just another flake in the mountain of letters you must receive, I'm attaching a bio I have used for consulting to give you some idea of who I am. I can also tell you that in a meeting with the Chair of the House Subcommittee on Health (US Congressman Joe Pitts) and the Leader of the Pennsylvania Senate (State Senator Dominic Pileggi), they and their staff were unable to refute a single point I made on this issue. In fact, their only push-back came in the form of a question of, "Why should I care if I can't pay?"--- My reply was simple. I said, "You are missing the point; you have no right to take it from me let alone to do it secretly." It was like sticking a pin in a balloon. Any and all argument simply collapsed.

A point of even greater interest was their full acceptance of my argument that the disclosure of this loss of access to care creates a whole new area of employer liability. In the past, employers could reasonably claim ignorance of the loss. However, given the release of my book "The Great Health Care Fraud", their excellent attorneys and the ERISA requirement to know and disclose their plans, employers will be facing very serious liability if they don't at least disclose this loss of access. However, since the loss stems from government action directly attached to the employer's plan on one hand and employers are solely responsible for the design of their plan on the other, I am not sure disclosure eliminates liability, particularly for self-insured companies like DuPont. After all, one could reasonably argue employers choose managed care plans specifically for their restricted access to care, i.e., lower cost. Furthermore, every subscriber of managed care insurance that has been denied coverage for necessary hospital care has also been denied the knowledge that the hospital was contractually required (the insurer's Provider Contract) to provide the denied care free of charge so long as the subscriber's doctor prescribed it.

Simply put, I sincerely believe the release of my book is a land mark event in that it exposes an unconstitutional fraud on the American people that goes to the very heart of what the Heritage Foundation is supposed to be about. And if Heritage is true to its stated mission, you will welcome this disclosure with open arms and use your extensive power and reach to enthusiastically spread the message contained in the book.

The last point I will make is that my ten (10) years in court against the insurance industry provides an excellent example of why our legal system is the best in the world. Misguided, underfunded and certainly ill-equipped for the fight, the system not only allowed this one small voice to prevail, but to resolve a wrong far too long hidden from the American people. --- A wrong that literally cost me and others the lives of those we loved.

Please see www.thegreathealthcarefraud.com and the book "The Great Health Care Fraud" at Amazon and Barnes and Noble. I would deeply appreciate receiving Heritage's position on the issue as well as your willingness to address this egregious affront to the law and the Constitution. And, of course, I stand ready to answer any question you may have on the issue.

Yours truly,

Frank Lobb

Appendix #4

Edwin J. Feulner's Letter to Author

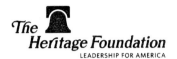

314 Massachusetts Avenue, NE
Washington, DC 20002-4999

(202) 546-4400
heritage.org

May 31, 2012

Mr. Frank H. Lobb
P.O. Box 242
Nottingham, PA 19362

Dear Mr. Lobb:

Thank you for your good letter of May 1, 2012.

I am in agreement with you: individuals should have full and complete control over their own health care dollars, and they should not be restricted in spending those dollars on the care that they determine is best for them.

Within the context of insurance, the reason why this is an issue at all is simple: individuals with health insurance do not own or control those policies in the same way that they own and control auto insurance, homeowners' or life insurance. For most Americans their employers own the policy.

This is not surprising. Employment-based coverage is almost exclusively favored by federal tax law, while those who purchase care independently can do so only with after-tax dollars. In effect, individual purchase of coverage is discouraged. So, today employers, as well as managed care officials and government officials, have more control over the flow of health care dollars than individuals. Much of that would change in the movement from a defined-benefit to defined-contribution financing of insurance, particularly if Congress does the right thing and provides tax relief for coverage directly to individuals regardless of where they work. This would give individuals direct control over the content of their policies. The Heritage Foundation has vigorously promoted this overarching reform for years.

Much of health insurance law and regulation remains within the jurisdiction of the states. I hasten to add, under our federal system, that is where it should remain. State laws vary widely in the regulation of insurance markets, as do state tort laws. In the case of Pennsylvania,

Mr. Frank H. Lobb
May 31, 2012   Page Two

if I understand your letter correctly, the state law governing health insurance contracts allowed for the restriction of employees in the purchase of medical services outside of the employer-based insurance, and it also exposed employers to liability for access restrictions.

I conferred with Dr. Moffit and he does indeed remember discussing your case with you several years ago when he was our Director of the Center for Health Policy. Since this was a matter of legal advice, he referred your case to Kent Masterson Brown, a nationally recognized expert in health insurance law and regulation, who had won a major suit against the Clinton Administration. It appears, however, that you have been successful in your litigation in Pennsylvania and the soundness of your position has been vindicated.

You are to be congratulated for your perseverance on this issue, as well as for the publication of your book. We do indeed have the best legal system in the world, as you say. It is a monument to the profound wisdom of the Founders and our peerless Constitution.

I wish you every success.

Sincerely,

Edwin J. Feulner
President

PS. In your letter you mentioned Dr. Jacques Chaouilli as a Canadian hero in the battle for health care freedom. In 2005, we published his Lecture, "A Victory for Freedom" (Heritage *Lecture* No. 892), a copy of which is attached. The lecture can also be found at www.heritage.org/research/healthcare/hl892.cfm .

Appendix #5

Author's Letter to U.S. Congressman Joe Pitts

Frank H. Lobb
P.O. Box 242
Nottingham, PA 19362

U. S. Congressman Joseph R. Pitts
150 North Queen Street, Suite 716
Lancaster, PA 17603

Feb. 20, 2013

Dear Congressman Pitts:

While the U. S. Supreme Court has held that we can't be denied the right to contribute to politicians and their campaigns, the nation's health care insurance industry has been allowed to strip my family and our employees of the right to pay for necessary and properly prescribed health care that our insurer "elects" to deny --- a fact you acknowledged in a meeting with Pennsylvania State Senator Dominic Pileggi and me some months back --- a meeting in which you also promised to respond to my request to testify before your House Subcommittee on Health.

Because I was denied the right to pay for the care prescribed for my wife and she died, I spent the better part of ten years suing our insurer for the details on how the nation's health care insurance industry has twisted the law and obfuscated their fiduciary duty in order to deny enrollees in managed care plans the right to pay for necessary health care when the insurer "elects" to deny care on the basis of cost or its own non-licensed medical opinion --- all carefully designed to overrule the opinion of an attending physician, circumvent well-established law, escape any direct responsibility, and deliver a stronger bottom line to the insurer. And, unlike Wendell Potter, this whistleblower is not bound by a confidentiality agreement with the insurance industry.

Simply put, the proof I have collected has been reviewed by the likes of The Heritage Foundation, the Cato Institute, attorneys at the Institute for Justice and any number of other attorneys specializing in health care and they have not found a single error of fact or law. Consequently, I just don't see how you can deny me the opportunity to testify without becoming complicit in hiding what can only be viewed as a blatantly unconstitutional denial of process and contract, an egregious fraud on the nation and a clear violation of the RICO Statute.

I have heard you speak passionately about the need to defend the Constitution and serve this great nation. And, like you, I consider myself a Conservative Republican and a strong advocate for private enterprise over government. So "PLEASE" allow me to testify on what I have learned. If I am wrong, your staff will be quick to set me straight --- nothing lost. However, since you have already acknowledged the basic point of my argument, as well as the all too real liability this creates for the nation's employers, I just don't see how a refusal to allow me to testify on this critical issue can be anything but a refusal to inform the American people as required under any number of laws and well held fiduciary responsibilities.

Please Congressman, help me raise this issue so that we can insure the individual freedom embodied in the Constitution remains available to every American --- especially in the pursuit of life itself!

Respectfully,

Frank H. Lobb

cc: State Senator Dominic Pileggi

Appendix #6

Author's 2nd Letter to Congressman Pitts

Frank H. Lobb
P.O. Box 242
Nottingham, PA 19362

U. S. Congressman Joseph R. Pitts
150 North Queen Street, Suite 716
Lancaster, PA 17603

Mar. 8, 2013

Dear Congressman Pitts:

Thank you for your fast and courteous response to my letter of Feb. 20, 2013. However, your letter has, quite honestly, left me confused. That said, let me respond to your questions one at a time.

1.) Your question as to whether the *"assertion"* in my letter is *"based on state law"* appears to ignore the fact that I met with you on two (2) separate occasions where you openly acknowledged the *"assertion"* is true and grounded in state laws that have been misapplied by insurers to <u>secretly</u> infringe an enrollee's right to contract and purchase health care.

2.) I have personally explained to you that I sued the Insurance Commissioner of the Commonwealth of Pennsylvania specifically because they refused to address the facts that you acknowledge are true --- an important source for the information I want to share through my testimony.

3.) This infringement of the right of contract and denial of process applies to all managed care plans. It has nothing to do with any particular company.

4.) Federal law has nothing to do with this issue except to make managed care insurers state actors and the hidden restrictions in managed care plans blatantly unconstitutional and, almost as certain, a violation of the fraud provisions in the Rico statute --- points no attorney I have spoken with has been able to refute.

Please remember that my second meeting with you included Pennsylvania State Senator Dominic Pileggi (a knowledgeable attorney), and you both acknowledged the facts as I have stated them as well as the very significant liability insurers have created for the nation's employers. And while I sincerely regret having to ask you to act against the interests of what we both know is an all-too-powerful insurance lobby, this is an issue that literally cost the life of my wife. Furthermore, if ten years of litigation taught me anything, it's the lengths the insurance industry is willing to go to keep these restrictions hidden. However, I just don't see myself having any other choice but to come to you for help. You are my Representative in Congress and someone I have voted for every time you have run in the belief that you are committed to doing the right thing for the people of your district and the country. You are also the Chair of the House Subcommittee on Health.

Let me again stress that I have heard you speak passionately about the need to defend the Constitution and the individual rights of the American people. And, like you, I consider myself a Conservative Republican and a strong advocate for private enterprise over government. So "PLEASE" allow me to testify on what I have learned. If I am wrong, your staff can set me straight --- nothing lost. However, since you have already acknowledged the basic point of my argument, as well as the misrepresentations that can be laid at the feet of the nation's managed care insurance industry, I just don't see how a refusal to allow me to testify can be anything but a refusal to inform the American people of the hidden restrictions in their managed care plans as required under any number of laws and well held fiduciary responsibilities.

Once again, PLEASE Congressman, help me raise this issue so that it can be discussed in the broad light of day. Help me insure that the individual freedom embodied in the Constitution remains available to every American --- especially in the pursuit of life itself!

And lastly, while I am not an attorney, I was deeply involved in the writing of The Clean Air Act and was credited with leading the effort that forced EPA to discard three years of work and redraft the compliance section of the Act around the instructions of Congress, presumptively credible evidence and my recommendations to Secretary Browner.

Respectfully,

Frank H. Lobb

cc: State Senator Dominic Pileggi

Appendix #7

Author's 3rd Letter to Congressman Pitts

Frank H. Lobb
P.O. Box 242
Nottingham, PA 19362

U. S. Congressman Joseph R. Pitts
150 North Queen Street, Suite 716
Lancaster, PA 17603

Mar. 16, 2013

Dear Congressman Pitts:

Once again, thank you for your fast reply to my letter and this time your request I call Tom Tillett in your Lancaster office to discuss the issue you and I have discussed on previous occasions. In order to insure Mr. Tillett and I begin on the same page, the issues are as follows:

1.) In order to control the cost of the care they promise, managed care insurance companies require doctors and hospitals to sign secret contracts that bar all forms of payment unless they support the insurer's decision on care. In other words, the "only" way an enrollee can get the care their insurer refuses to approve, is for the doctor and hospital to knowingly agree to provide the care free of charge ---- all under color of state action. It's as unconstitutional as it can get as well as a deliberate fraud, tortious interference with contract, a violation of the covenant of good faith and fair dealing, the Hobbs Act and the RICO Statutes.

2.) You have acknowledged the above facts are true.

3.) I have repeatedly requested to testify before your Subcommittee on Health.

4.) You have promised to respond to my request to testify.

Respectfully,

Frank H. Lobb

cc: State Senator Dominic Pileggi

Appendix #8

Representative Provider Contract

The following is a representative Provider Contract without its mundane boilerplate provisions. It is not a copy of any specific insurer's provider contract to avoid the charge of disclosing secret proprietary information. However, it is an accurate representation the provider contracts insurance companies use to restrict the freedom of doctors and hospitals to deliver appropriate care to enrollees while empowering the insurance company's ability to deny both care and coverage.

....

THIS PARTICIPATING PROVIDER AGREEMENT ("Agreement"), is made and entered into between **INSURER** and **HOSPITAL/DOCTOR** to establish terms and conditions for the rendering and payment of services to Subscribers in accordance with insurance plans issued by **INSURER**.

NOW, THEREFORE, in consideration of the premises and mutual covenants contained herein and other good and valuable consideration, the receipt and sufficiency of which are hereby acknowledged, it is mutually agreed by and between the Parties as follows:

ARTICLE 1

DEFINITIONS

For the purpose of this Agreement, the following definitions shall apply:

1.1 CHARGES – The Hospital's/Doctor's itemized listing of the rates it charges for patient services.
1.2 COVERED SERVICES – The services listed in a Subscriber's insurance benefit package AND rendered to the Subscriber.
1.3 NON-COVERED SERVICES – The services that are defined as NOT available services in the Subscriber's insurance Plan and benefit package (typically limited to elective cosmetic surgery and experimental treatments).
1.4 NETWORK – The participating providers with which Insurer, its affiliates, contractors and subcontractors has contracted to furnish COVERED SERVICES under a subscriber benefit package issued by Insurer.
1.5 ENROLLEE – A subscriber who is eligible to receive COVERED SERVICES under an insurance Plan and benefit package issued by Insurer.
1.6 SUBSCRIBER – An enrolled and eligible individual, or dependents, who has satisfied the criteria for benefits under an insurance Plan provided and administered by Insurer.
1.7 EMERGENCY – A sudden onset of acute medical or psychiatric symptoms of sufficient severity, that in the absence of immediate medical attention, could result in: 1.) Permanent injury to the subscriber, or 2.) Cause other serious medical or psychologi-

cal consequences.

1.8 EMERGENCY CARE – Medically necessary care and services and supplies provided to a subscriber in an emergency.

1.9 MEDICALLY NECESSARY or APPROPRIATE CARE – The requirement that Covered Services are required, in the opinion of: (1.) the primary care physician, or the referred specialist, as applicable, consistent with Insurer's policies, coverage requirements and utilization guidelines; and (2.) Insurer, in order to diagnose and treat a subscriber, as applicable, and:

a. Are provided in accordance with established standards and practices;
b. Are required to improve the subscriber's health and health outcome; and
c. Are as cost-effective as any available and approved alternative.

SECTION 2. PROVISION of COVERED SERVICES

2.1 Hospital/Doctor shall furnish Medically Necessary or Appropriate Services to eligible Subscribers in accordance with the terms and conditions of the Subscriber's insurance Plan and this Agreement.

2.2 Hospital/Doctor shall be solely responsible for the quality of Covered Services rendered to Subscriber. Hospital/Doctor further acknowledges that any action taken by Insurer pursuant to utilization management or cost containment in no way absolves Hospital/Doctor of the responsibility to provide appropriate care to Subscriber.

2.3 Covered Services shall be rendered a Subscriber by Hospital/Doctor without any advance deposit or other charge to Subscriber, except for copayments and deductible payments described in the Subscriber's insurance Plan.

2.4 Doctor/Hospital agrees to render Covered Services in accordance with: (a) all terms and conditions set forth in this Agreement, (b) all applicable laws and regulations, and (c) the same manner and timeliness as all other patients without regard to reimbursement.

SECTION 3. PAYMENT for SERVICES RENDERED

3.1 Hospital/Doctor shall submit claims for Covered Services no more than 90 days from the date the Covered Services are rendered.

3.2 Insurer shall pay Hospital/Doctor in accordance with the rates set herein for Medically Necessary and Appropriate Covered Services rendered Subscribers per the terms and conditions set forth in this Agreement.

3.3 Covered Services approved by Insurer and rendered by Hospital/Doctor shall be paid as provided herein, UNLESS: (a) excluded as a Non-Covered Service by a Subscribers insurance Plan and benefit package, (b) Insurer informs Hospital/Doctor that a given service is not a Covered Service, or (c) Insurer determines the service to be not Medically Necessary or Appropriate.

3.4 If all or any part of the Covered Services rendered a Subscriber by Hospital/Doctor was not ordered by a properly licensed health professional operating within the scope of that license, the Hospital/Doctor shall not bill or charge either Insurer or the Subscriber for that portion of the Covered Service.

3.5 Hospital/Doctor shall accept payments made by Insurer for Covered Services, including non-payment, as payment in full for all Covered Services rendered to a Subscriber and shall comply with the Employee Hold Harmless provision set forth below. The Insurer's payment, including non-payment, shall therefore discharge all obligation of Subscriber for Covered Services.

3.6   In the event Insurer makes an incorrect payment or an overpayment to Hospital/ Doctor, Hospital/Doctor agrees to refund or reimburse such amounts within five (5) business days. If Hospital/Doctor fails to refund or reimburse an overpayment, Hospital/Doctor hereby authorizes Insurer to withhold or offset future payments against amounts owed Hospital/Doctor.

SECTION 4. BILLING

4.1   Hospital/Doctor agree to submit bills to Insurer for Covered Services by the later of: (a) ninety days following the date Insurer issues billing approval to Hospital/ Doctor or (2) ninety days following the last day of the calendar year in which the Subscriber was discharged from the hospital or ended treatment. If Hospital/Doctor fails to submit billing within this defined period, Insurer shall not be responsible for payment for those Covered Services and Hospital/Doctor shall not bill Subscriber for those Covered Services.

4.2   Insurer agrees to exercise its best efforts to pay appropriate claims for Covered Services within thirty (30) days of receipt of such claims.

SECTION 5. UTILIZATION REVIEW

5.1   All Covered Services rendered to Subscriber by Hospital/Doctor are subject to a medical and utilization review by Insurer or its designee.

5.2   Hospital/Doctor shall notify Insurer of all elective inpatient care to be rendered to a subscriber prior to admission or rendering such elective care.

5.3   Hospital/Doctor shall notify Insurer of all emergency admissions of Subscribers within one (1) business day of such admission.

5.4   Hospital/Doctor shall pre-certify all non-emergency admissions of Subscribers prior to admission by obtaining Insurer's approval of the Medical Necessity or Appropriateness of the admission and proposed length of stay.

5.5   Hospital/Doctor agrees Insurer shall not approve an inpatient admission until all necessary information is provided Insurer.

5.6   Where pre-certification is required but not performed, any and all services and days of care rendered prior to Insurer's pre-certification and approval shall not be billed or charged to Insurer or Subscriber.

5.7   Hospital/Doctor agrees Insurer shall review the Medical Necessity or Appropriateness of an inpatient admission or course of treatment on a daily basis and free to find such admission or course of treatment not Medically Necessary or Appropriate.

5.8   Whenever the Insurer's review of Medically Necessary or Appropriate determines a particular inpatient admission or course of treatment is not Medically Necessary or Appropriate, Hospital/Doctor shall not bill or charge Insurer or Subscriber for that denied stay or treatment. Hospital/Doctor further agrees such reviews and denials can be retroactive and reverse earlier approvals by Insurer or Insurer's designee.

5.9   Whenever an admission or some portion of an admission is determined by Insurer to be not Medically Necessary or Appropriate or other requirements set forth herein are not met, the entire admission shall be denied and the Hospital/Doctor shall not bill or charge Insurer or Subscriber for any services associated with such denied stay or treatment.

5.10   Should Insurer determine a requested admission or course of treatment is not Medically Necessary or Appropriate and Hospital/Doctor nonetheless provides that admission or course of treatment, Hospital/Doctor shall not bill or charge Insurer or Subscriber for any related costs associated with that denied admission or treatment.

SECTION 6. EMPLOYEE HOLD HARMLESS

6.1   Hospital/Doctor agrees that in no event, including but not limited to non-payment by Insurer, Insurer's insolvency or breach of this Agreement, shall Hospital/Doctor, one of its subcontractors, or any of its employees or independent contractors bill, charge, collect a deposit from, seek compensation, remuneration or reimbursement from, or have any recourse against a Subscriber, or persons other than Insurer acting on behalf for services provided pursuant to this Agreement. This provision shall not prohibit the collection of coinsurance, copayments or charges for non-Covered Services. Hospital/Doctor further agrees that (1) this provision shall survive the termination of this Agreement regardless of the cause giving rise to the termination and shall be construed to be for the benefit of the Subscriber, and that (2) this provision supersedes any oral or written contrary agreement now existing or hereinafter entered into between Hospital/Doctor and Subscriber or persons acting on their behalf.

SECTION 7. CONFIDENTIALITY AND DISCLOSURE

7.1   Hospital/Doctor agree not to disclose any information pertaining to business conducted by Insurer, including, but not limited to the payments for Covered Services. Hospital/Doctor further agrees that all such information shall be considered confidential and proprietary and unless required by law, shall not be disclosed, except as otherwise approved by written consent of Insurer.

7.2   Hospital/Doctor specifically acknowledge and agree that a breach of the foregoing provisions will cause Insurer irreparable harm and that the remedy at law for any such breach will be inadequate and that Insurer, in addition to any other relief available to it, shall be entitled to equitable relief and temporary and permanent injunctive relief without the necessity of proving actual damages or posting any bond whatsoever.

SECTION 8. INDEMNIFICATION

8.1.1   Hospital/Doctor agrees to indemnify and hold harmless Insurer from any suit, cost, claim or expense, including, but not limited to, the cost of defense incurred by Insurer as a result of negligent actions or breach of this Agreement by Hospital/Doctor or their employees, contractors or subcontractors in connection with rendering

Covered Services pursuant to this Agreement.

SECTION 9. TERM

9.1 This Agreement shall commence as of the date hereof and shall continue for three (3) years, and thereafter shall automatically renew for successive terms of one (1) year. Notwithstanding the foregoing, this Agreement shall not be effective until approved by State Department of Insurance/Health.

SECTION 10. TERMINATION

10.1 Either party may terminate this Agreement by providing the other party with not less than 60 days prior written notice.

10.2 Insurer may immediately terminate this Agreement if, in its sole opinion, Hospital/Doctor fails to comply with any Insurer Policies or Procedures and such failure would reasonably have a material adverse effect on Insurer.

10.3 Insurer may immediately terminate this Agreement if, in its sole opinion, Hospital/Doctor are in breach of any portion of this Agreement and failed to cure such Breach within 30 days of written notification by insurer.

10.4 In the event Hospital/Doctor is providing services to a Subscriber as of the date of termination of this Agreement, Hospital/Doctor shall continue to furnish those services and facilities contemplated to that Subscriber and all other Subscribers who were receiving such services on the date of termination. Hospital's/Doctor's right to receive reimbursement for such Covered Services shall continue to be governed by the applicable terms of this Agreement. This provision shall survive the termination of this Agreement for any reason.

SECTION 11. APPEAL OF UTILIZATION REVIEW DETERMINATIONS

11.1 Hospital/Doctor has the right to appeal an adverse determination by Insurer or its designee on the Medical Necessity or Appropriateness of any requested inpatient admission, length of stay or course of treatment.

11.2 Hospital/Doctor agree to comply with Insurer's policies, procedures and all final determinations of appropriate care and coverage

11.3 Hospital/Doctor agrees decisions by the Insurer's Appeals Panel shall be final, binding and non-appealable for all parties.

IN WITNESS WHEREOF, the undersigned have executed this Agreement on the date set forth below.

INSURANCE COMPANY   HOSPITAL/DOCTOR

By: _____   By: _____

Date_____   Date _____

Appendix #9

Sample Enrollee Reply to a Hospital Bill

From: Managed Care Enrollee
To: Hospital Billing Office
Subject: My right to understand the bill I just received

Date

      I have received your bill and need to remind you that the law and the provider contract that you have signed with my insurance company severely limit what you can bill me, regardless of any failure of my insurance company to pay for my care. Furthermore, because: 1.) Your bill is computed from a long list of individually coded and priced items taken from what I believe you refer to as your Chargemaster, 2.) I have a right to the prices for each of these items that are listed in the provider contract that you have signed with my insurance company, 3.) My insurance company has the authority to deny or bundle any and all of your individual charges in order to reduce the overall amount of your bill, 4.) Any individual charge or group of charges that my insurance company elects to deny, for whatever reason, cannot be billed to me nor can it be used in computing any co-insurance, deductible or cap, 5.) The application of any co-insurance, deductible or cap requires a detailed explanation of items 1 through 4 as well as information you can only obtain from my insurance company, and 6.) Any appeal of my insurance company's denial of charges, bundling and/or failures to pay for whatever reason is solely your responsibility. Consequently, I am requesting the following information as the minimum needed to understand your bill.

1. A complete list of the individual items, codes and prices from your Chargemasted that comprise your bill.
2. The discounted prices listed in your provider contract for each of these same items.
3. My insurance company's decisions on whether to pay for "each" of these same items, including any bundling of charges.
4. A detailed accounting of how my insurance company's decisions on payment affect any applicable co-insurance, deductible and/or cap.
5. A copy of the Enrollee Hold Harmless Clause in your provider contract that defines what you can and cannot bill me.
6. A copy of all other provisions and language in your provider contract that limit what you can bill me.
7. The same above information (1 through 6) for my secondary insurance, when and where applicable.

Because the information I am requesting is no more than: 1.) what is needed to understand your bill, 2.) what your publication on patients' rights and responsibilities promises and 3.) what the law entitles me to receive; I have to assume it is readily available. If I am wrong or you have a different understanding of any of my above statements or requests, please get back to me. For like you, I want to get you properly paid and to put this matter behind me.

Sincerely,

One Confused Enrollee

Attachment #10

Medicare Notification of Possible Noncoverage

A. Notifier:

B. Patient Name: **C. Identification Number:**

Advance Beneficiary Notice of Noncoverage (ABN)

NOTE: If Medicare doesn't pay for **D.** _____ below, you may have to pay.
Medicare does not pay for everything, even some care that you or your health care provider have good reason to think you need. We expect Medicare may not pay for the **D.** _____ below.

D.	E. Reason Medicare May Not Pay:	F. Estimated Cost

WHAT YOU NEED TO DO NOW:
- Read this notice, so you can make an informed decision about your care.
- Ask us any questions that you may have after you finish reading.
- Choose an option below about whether to receive the **D.** _____ listed above.
  Note: If you choose Option 1 or 2, we may help you to use any other insurance that you might have, but Medicare cannot require us to do this.

G. OPTIONS: Check only one box. We cannot choose a box for you.

☐ **OPTION 1.** I want the **D.** _____ listed above. You may ask to be paid now, but I also want Medicare billed for an official decision on payment, which is sent to me on a Medicare Summary Notice (MSN). I understand that if Medicare doesn't pay, I am responsible for payment, but **I can appeal to Medicare** by following the directions on the MSN. If Medicare does pay, you will refund any payments I made to you, less co-pays or deductibles.

☐ **OPTION 2.** I want the **D.** _____ listed above, but do not bill Medicare. You may ask to be paid now as I am responsible for payment. **I cannot appeal if Medicare is not billed**.

☐ **OPTION 3.** I don't want the **D.** _____ listed above. I understand with this choice I am **not** responsible for payment, and **I cannot appeal to see if Medicare would pay.**

H. Additional Information:

This notice gives our opinion, not an official Medicare decision. If you have other questions on this notice or Medicare billing, call **1-800-MEDICARE** (1-800-633-4227/**TTY:** 1-877-486-2048).
Signing below means that you have received and understand this notice. You also receive a copy.

I. Signature:	J. Date:

According to the Paperwork Reduction Act of 1995, no persons are required to respond to a collection of information unless it displays a valid OMB control number. The valid OMB control number for this information collection is 0938-0566. The time required to complete this information collection is estimated to average 7 minutes per response, including the time to review instructions, search existing data resources, gather the data needed, and complete and review the information collection. If you have comments concerning the accuracy of the time estimate or suggestions for improving this form, please write to: CMS, 7500 Security Boulevard, Attn: PRA Reports Clearance Officer, Baltimore, Maryland 21244-1850.

Form CMS-R-131 (03/11)   Form Approved OMB No. 0938-0566

Attachment #11

HMO Model Act
National Association of Insurance Commissioners
(as recently modified)

Section 19.   Enrollee Hold Harmless Clause for Covered Persons

A.) Except for coinsurance, deductibles or copayments as specifically provided in the evidence of coverage, in no event, including but not limited to nonpayment by the health maintenance organization, insolvency of the health maintenance organization or breach of contract among the health maintenance organization, risk bearing entity or participating provider bill, charge, collect a deposit from, seek compensation, remuneration or reimbursement from, or have any recourse against a covered person or a person (other than the health maintenance organization) acting on the behalf of the covered person for covered services provided. No risk bearing entity or participating provider, nor any agent, trustee or assignee of the risk bearing entity or participating provider may maintain an action at law against a covered person to collect sums owed by the health maintenance organization.

B.) All contracts among health maintenance organizations, risk bearing entities, and participating providers shall include a hold harmless provision specifying protection for covered persons. Any attempted waiver or amendment in a matter materially adverse to the interests of covered persons of a hold harmless provision shall be null and void and unenforceable.

C.) The requirement of Subsection B shall be met by including a provision substantially similar to the following:

> Provider agrees that in no event, including but not limited to nonpayment by the health maintenance organization or intermediary organization, insolvency of the health maintenance organization or intermediary organization, or breach of this agreement shall the provider bill, charge, collect a deposit from, seek compensation, remuneration or reimbursement from, or have any recourse against a covered person or a person (other than the health maintenance organization or intermediary organization) acting on behalf of the covered person for covered services provided pursuant to this agreement. This agreement does not prohibit the provider from collecting coinsurance, deductibles copayments or services in excess of limits, as specifically provided in the evidence of coverage, or fees for uncovered services delivered on a fee-for-service basis to covered persons.

D.) (1)   Any statement to a covered person shall clearly state the amounts billed to the health maintenance organization and include a notice explaining that covered persons are not responsible for amounts owed by the health maintenance organization.

(2) All contracts among health maintenance organizations, risk bearing entities, amd participating providers shall require that all statements sent to covered persons clearly state the amounts billed to the health maintenance organization and include a notice explaining that covered persons are not responsible for amounts owed by the health maintenance organization.

(3) The notice requirements in this section shall be met by including in the statement to covered persons a provision substantially similar to the following:

"Notice: You are not responsible for any amounts owed by your health maintenance organization."

E.) Any violation of the provisions of this section shall constitute an unfair trade practice pursuant to [insert reference to state insurance fraud statute] and shall subject the health care provider to monitory penalties in accordance with [insert reference to state insurance fraud statute] and notification to the [insert reference to appropriate licensing entity for type of provider].

Drafting Comments:

a.) States that do not authorize insurance departments to take actions against providers should not adopt Subsection E and should consider other options such as contacting the state attorney general's office or other appropriate state official.

b.) States with consumer protection acts that provide covered persons with a private right of action should consider including a reference in Subsection E.

Author's Note:

The above is what the Author believes is an accurate depiction of the language used by the National Association of Insurance Commissioners to update their HMO Model ACT in 2003. It is not, nor is it represented as an exact "reprint" of that material.

Appendix 12

Letters to U. S. Senators Coburn, Hatch & Burr

The following two letters were sent to each of the above three U. S Senators to congratulate them on their joint announcement of a Republican plan to replace Obamacare. I will argue that their failure to provide any reply what-so-ever to my letters speaks volumes on how deeply committed my Republican Party is to protecting the managed-care insurance industry along with their hidden power to ration health care. I will also argue that it is even a greater indication of their fear over the threat that Obamacare with its individual mandate poses for the insurance industry and their use of the Enrollee Hold harmless clause. After all, these Senators could have simply thanked me for my letter and interest in health care reform. They could have done what they always do and replied with a form letter and a stamped copy of the senator's signature. So simple and yet complete silence from all three U. S. Senators.

A conspiracy? You bet it is. Just as the Chief of Staff for U. S. Congressman Joe Pitts told me in no uncertain and heated terms, *"You can forget about testifying."*

Frank H. Lobb
P.O. Box 242
Nottingham, PA 19362

U. S. Senator Coburn/Hatch/Burr
Senate Office Building
Washington, DC 20510

March 7, 2014

Dear Senator:
Congratulations on your proposed legislation to replace Obamacare, most particularly,
Title 5, Section 501 of the proposal that *"requires"* the disclosure of *"coverage details."*
My question is, does this proposed transparency include informing the American people
that they secretly surrender the "right" to self-pay for care their insurer refuses to cover
when they get health insurance. The only permitted exception is for elective cosmetic
care.

The Chair of the House Subcommittee on Health, U. S. Congressman Joe Pitts, has
acknowledged this loss on two separate occasions that I pursued the issue with him.
However, he has absolutely refused to make the information public. He has also refused
to allow me to testify on this outrageous loss of freedom and due process.

Please understand that this issue is particularly important to me as I was refused the
right to pay for my wife's care. She died while I fought to understand how an insurance
company could deny me the right to pay for care that was prescribed by our doctor as
absolutely necessary and I was willing to pay for in advance. So when I say enrollees in
managed care plans are secretly stripped of their right to purchase necessary health care
their insurer, for whatever reason, refuses to approve, I am not making some wild and
unsubstantiated claim. I have the hard documented proof as well as my congressman's,
Congressman Pitt's, acknowledgement of this undisclosed loss.

Given your reputation for honesty and straight talk together with the importance of my
question, I assume we can both agree that anything less than an in depth and responsible
response to this letter can only be an attempt to join Congressman Pitts in keeping this
critical *"coverage detail"* from the American people --- something your proposed legislation and our Republican Party claim to be adamantly against.

Very Respectfully,

Frank H. Lobb

cc: Matthew Herper, Forbes Magazine
        Mary Agnes Carey, Kaiser Health News
        Karl Stark, Philadelphia Inquirer

Frank H. Lobb
P.O. Box 242
Nottingham, PA 19362

U. S. Senator Coburn/Hatch/Burr
Senate Office Building
Washington, DC 20510

May 14, 2014

Dear Senator:

More than 2 months ago I sent you the attached letter and have received nothing in reply. Consequently, as disappointed as I may be, your silence confirms that, like Congressman Pitts, you are in the camp of those refusing to disclose the loss of our right to self-pay for any prescribed necessary health care that our insurer denies along with the accompanying loss of our personal and private doctor-patient relationship. These are two losses that cannot be denied and ones that MUST be disclosed in order to comply with existing law and fiduciary duties.

It blows my mind that you, along with other leaders of my party, would promise full transparency in replacing Obamacare, but support hiding the impact of the Enrollee Hold Harmless clause on health insurance. I honestly thought you and our party were better than this!

Frank H. Lobb

cc: Matthew Herper, Forbes Magazine
       Mary Agnes Carey, Kaiser Health News
       Karl Stark, Philadelphia Inquirer

Appendix 13

The following correspondence with U. S. Senator John McCain provides a great way to end the book. It provides the perfect example of why we can't look to Washington or my Republican Party for honest answers when it comes to health care.

My letter to Senator McCain was sent on September 16, 2013. It simply asked for help in disclosing what U. S. Congressman Joe Pitts (the Chair of The House Subcommittee on Health) had acknowledged but refused to disclose to the American people, i.e., the truth about our health care system's fraudulent rationing and billing practices. Ten months later, Senator McCain responds without even addressing my request for help and arguing for changes in the health care system that he has to know are absolutely false on their face and nothing more than a political smoke-screen for the managed care insurance industry.

1.) Allowing the purchase of health insurance across state lines would necessitate placing the federal government in charge of regulating health care and insurance, an authority that has been specifically assigned to the states and one that Republicans will never agree to change. See Appendix 4, Edwin J. Feulner's, President of The Heritage Foundation, letter.

2.) Claiming that we should simply pursue *"common sense reforms that will drive down the cost of care"* is a grossly simplistic claim for an unbelievably complex problem. It's a claim that absolutely ignores the realities of the health care market — a market where competition is essentially impossible because of the regional monopolies that have been created with the support of the Republican Party, and where the insurance industry contractually bars the disclosure the pricing an enrollee is entitled to receive (the industry's *"privately"* negotiate pricing for a particular plan and provider).

Appendix 14

Author's Letter to Senator McCain

Frank H. Lobb
P. O. Box 242
Nottingham, PA 19362
Phone: (610) 932-8488
e-Mail: frank.lobb@kennett.net

U. S. Senator John McCain
2201 East Camelback Rd., Suite 115
Phoenix, AZ 85016

Sep 16, 2013

Dear Senator McCain:

This morning on the Morning Joe program you gave an excellent defense of the need "to do what is right for the Country." As a retired Navy pilot, like you, I feel we have both made this an inseparable part of who we are. Consequently, I am asking for your help in a matter that unfairly causes suffering, death and fraudulent billing practices in our nation's health care system on a daily basis. --- An issue the politicians in my state refuse to touch.

Well hidden in the laws of every state is a provision that bars doctors and hospitals from billing anyone with health insurance for care their insurer refuses to approve. The only exception is for elective cosmetic surgery. In essence, the only way my doctor and hospital can render care that my insurer refuses to approve is to render it free of charge --- even if I offer to write a check on the spot to cover the cost.

As crazy as this may sound, I have the documented proof as well as the acknowledgement of Congressman Joe Pitts, Chair of the House Subcommittee on Health (the Representative for my District). I was also personally refused the right to pay for my wife's care. To quote Congressman Pitts, "Why should I care if I can't pay for health care?"

Please Senator, help me disclose this unreasonable bar on the right to privately contract for necessary health care --- a disclosure required by federal law or, at least, take the time to explain where I am wrong on the facts or the law. I will be more than willing to come to Washington to discuss this important issue with you or your staff.

Sincerely,

Frank H. Lobb

cc: Mary Agnes Carey, Kaiser Health News

Attach the scanned copy of John McCain's Jul 3, 2014 letter to me.

Appendix 15

Senator McCain's Letter to Frank Lobb

JOHN McCAIN
ARIZONA

COMMITTEE ON ARMED SERVICES

COMMITTEE ON HEALTH,
EDUCATION, LABOR, AND PENSIONS

COMMITTEE ON HOMELAND SECURITY
AND GOVERNMENTAL AFFAIRS

COMMITTEE ON INDIAN AFFAIRS

United States Senate

241 RUSSELL SENATE OFFICE BUILDING
WASHINGTON, DC 20510-0303
(202) 224-2235

2201 EAST CAMELBACK ROAD
SUITE 115
PHOENIX, AZ 85016
(602) 952-2410

122 NORTH CORTEZ STREET
SUITE 108
PRESCOTT, AZ 86301
(928) 445-0833

407 WEST CONGRESS STREET
SUITE 103
TUCSON, AZ 85701
(520) 670-6334

TELEPHONE FOR HEARING IMPAIRED
(602) 952-0170

July 3, 2014

Frank H. Lobb
PO Box 242
Nottingham, PA 19362-0242

Dear Friend,

Thank you for contacting me with your views on the health reform legislation passed by Congress in 2010.

Three years after its passage, the Patient Protection and Affordable Care Act (PPACA) remains one of the most controversial bills ever considered in Congress. While I support improving our health care delivery system to bring down costs and increase access to affordable health insurance, and have put forth several detailed proposals, the PPACA is not the answer. As written, this legislation would lead to higher health care costs, increased taxes, trillions of dollars in new federal spending, $715 billion in cuts to Medicare, and more expensive health insurance.

Despite the President's repeated claims to the contrary, the new unsustainable entitlement created by PPACA will add to the deficit, undermine America's global leadership in health care innovation and quality of care, and put the federal government in charge of writing the health insurance policies that individuals and employers are mandated to purchase.

I believe we need to repeal the new health care law and replace it with common sense reforms that will drive down the cost of care while improving accessibility to affordable health insurance coverage.

This can be achieved by increasing choice and competition by allowing individuals to purchase insurance policies across state lines, enacting medical malpractice reform, focusing on prevention and incentivizing wellness programs, and establishing affordable coverage mechanisms for individuals with high-risk and preexisting conditions.

I will continue my efforts to replace the unsustainable health reform law that was forced through Congress with reforms based on competition and freedom rather than the expansion of the federal bureaucracy.

Thank you again for writing to me. Please feel free to contact me if you have any other comments or questions.

Sincerely,

John McCain
United States Senator

JM/JS

CPSIA information can be obtained at www.ICGtesting.com
Printed in the USA
LVOW12s0919100515

437936LV00023B/862/P